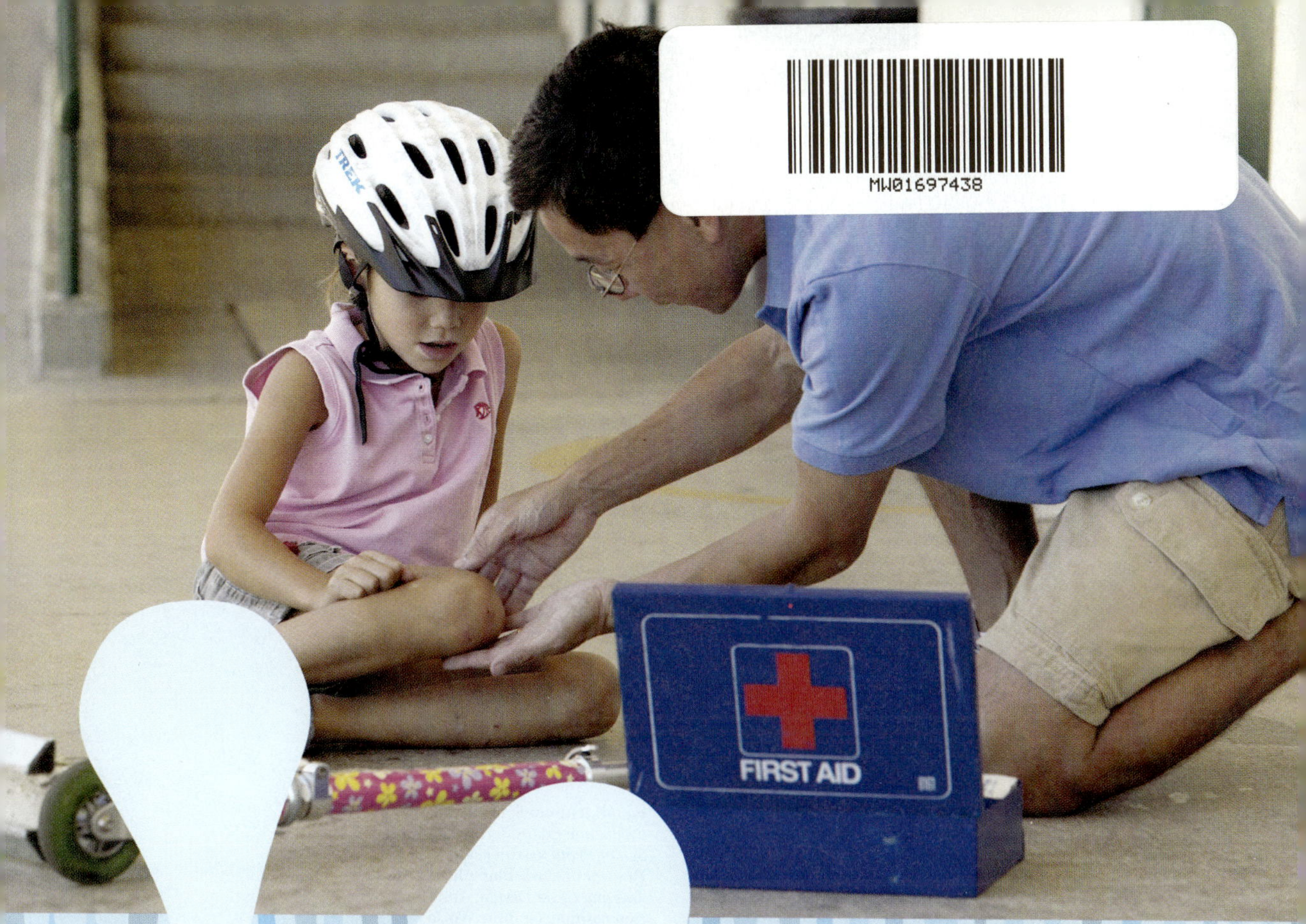

Pediatric First Aid for Caregivers and Teachers

American Academy of Pediatrics
DEDICATED TO THE HEALTH OF ALL CHILDREN™

JONES & BARTLETT LEARNING

World Headquarters
Jones & Bartlett Learning
5 Wall Street
Burlington, MA 01803
978-443-5000
info@jbpub.com
www.jbpub.com

Jones and Bartlett's books and products are available through most bookstores and online booksellers. To contact Jones and Bartlett Publishers directly, call 800-832-0034, fax 978-443-8000, or visit our website www.jbpub.com.

Substantial discounts on bulk quantities of Jones and Bartlett's publications are available to corporations, professional associations, and other qualified organizations. For details and specific discount information, contact the special sales department at Jones and Bartlett via the above contact information or send an email to specialsales@jbpub.com.

American Academy of Pediatrics

DEDICATED TO THE HEALTH OF ALL CHILDREN™

Managing Editor:
Thaddeus Anderson, Manager, Life Support Programs-Revised First Edition
Jodi Turner, Manager, Life Support Programs-First Edition

Ellen Buerk, MD, MEd, FAAP, AAP Board Reviewer
Robert Perelman, MD, FAAP, Director, Department of Education
Wendy Simon, MA, CAE, Director, Life Support Programs
Eileen Schoen, Manager, Life Support Programs
Kristy Goddyn, Life Support Records Assistant
Bonnie Molnar, Life Support Assistant
Tina Patel, Life Support Assistant
Kimberly Liotus, Division Coordinator

American Academy of Pediatrics
141 Northwest Point Boulevard
Post Office Box 927
Elk Grove Village, IL 60009-0927
847-434-4798
www.aap.org

Production Credits
Chief Executive Officer: Clayton E. Jones
Chief Operating Officer: Donald W. Jones, Jr.
President, Higher Education and Professional Publishing: Robert W. Holland, Jr.
V.P., Sales and Marketing: William J. Kane
V.P., Production and Design: Anne Spencer
V.P., Manufacturing and Inventory Control: Therese Connell
Publisher, Public Safety Group: Kimberly Brophy
Publisher, Emergency Care: Lawrence Newell
Editor: Jennifer S. Kling
Production Editor: Jenny L. McIsaac
Senior Photo Researcher: Kimberly Potvin
Director of Marketing: Alisha Weisman
Text and Cover Design: Anne Spencer
Composition: Graphic World
Cover Photograph: © David Young-Wolff/PhotoEdit
Text Printing and Binding: Courier Company
Cover Printing: Courier Company

The Academy and Jones and Bartlett Publishers would like to thank the following reviewers: Linda Gosselin, Linda Lipinsky, Eileen Schoen, Wendy Simon, Charles Stanzione, and Judith Tanner.

The procedures in this text are based on the most current recommendations of responsible sources. The publisher and the Academy make no guarantee as to, and assume no responsibility for the correctness, sufficiency, or completeness of such information or recommendations. Other or additional safety measures may be required under particular circumstances. This text is intended solely as a guide to the appropriate procedures to be employed when providing first aid. It is not intended as a statement of the procedures required in any particular situation, because circumstances can vary widely from one situation to another.

The American Academy of Pediatrics reserves the right to disclose personal information of course participants/providers for administrative purposes such as to verify participation or classes taken or to validate the status of any course completion card. In no event shall the American Academy of Pediatrics or the publisher have any liability for disclosure or use of information for such purposes or responsibility for the consequences of any actions in reliance on such information.

Library of Congress Cataloging-in-Publication Data Not Available at Time of Printing

ISBN: 978-1-4496-7386-4

6048

Additional photo credits appear on page 311, which constitutes a continuation of the copyright page.

Printed in the United States of America
15 14 13 12 11 10 9 8 7 6 5 4

American Academy of Pediatrics

DEDICATED TO THE HEALTH OF ALL CHILDREN™

Dear Caregivers and Teachers:

As a caregiver or teacher, you have the important task of nurturing and providing care for children. A critical aspect of caring for children includes maintaining a safe and healthy environment. Learning first aid skills is an important step in ensuring a secure environment for those children in your care.

On behalf of the Board of Directors of the American Academy of Pediatrics, I am pleased to introduce a quality educational program: *Pediatric First Aid for Caregivers and Teachers* (PedFACTs). This exciting program is designed specifically to prepare caregivers and teachers to appropriately recognize and respond to the ill or injured child.

It is the mission of the American Academy of Pediatrics to attain optimal physical, mental and social health and well-being for all infants, children, adolescents and young adults. To support this mission, the goal of the PedFACTs Steering Committee is to provide a first aid program that will enhance and expand the knowledge and skills of those who care for children. I applaud the efforts of the many dedicated individuals who participated in the development of the PedFACTs materials.

I would also like to thank you personally for your dedication to caring for children. Working together we really can make a difference.

Sincerely,

Errol R Alden, MD, FAAP
Executive Director/CEO
American Academy of Pediatrics

Contents

Resource Preview

Pediatric First Aid for Caregivers and Teachers

The American Academy of Pediatrics (AAP) is pleased to bring you Pediatric First Aid for Caregivers and Teachers (PedFACTs), a new national pediatric first aid course.

The PedFACTs course is designed to give teachers and caregivers the education and confidence that they need to effectively care for children. This participant manual is the core of the PedFACTs program with features that will reinforce and expand on the essential information.

Each topic is divided into three sections:

1. **What You Should Know,** providing background information
2. **What You Should Look For,** providing assessment information
3. **What You Should Do,** providing first aid treatment information

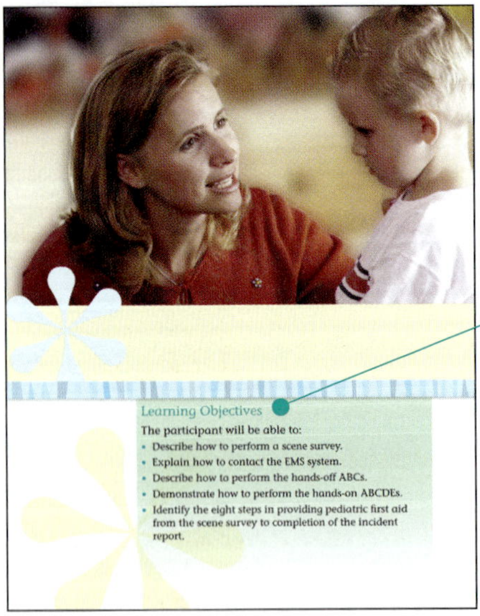

Learning Objectives

Learning objectives are placed at the beginning of each topic to highlight what students should learn on that topic.

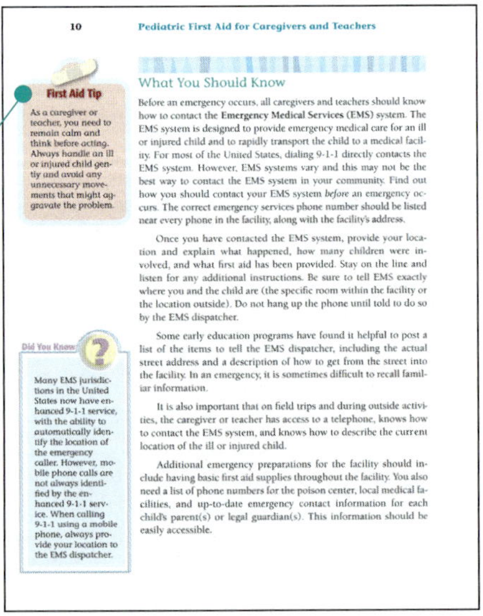

10 Pediatric First Aid for Caregivers and Teachers

First Aid Tip

As a caregiver or teacher, you need to remain calm and think before acting. Always handle an ill or injured child gently and avoid any unnecessary movements that might aggravate the problem.

What You Should Know

Before an emergency occurs, all caregivers and teachers should know how to contact the **Emergency Medical Services (EMS)** system. The EMS system is designed to provide emergency medical care for an ill or injured child and to rapidly transport the child to a medical facility. For most of the United States, dialing 9-1-1 directly contacts the EMS system. However, EMS systems vary and this may not be the best way to contact the EMS system in your community. Find out how you should contact your EMS system *before* an emergency occurs. The correct emergency services phone number should be listed near every phone in the facility, along with the facility's address.

Once you have contacted the EMS system, provide your location and explain what happened, how many children were involved, and what first aid has been provided. Stay on the line and listen for any additional instructions. Be sure to tell EMS exactly where you and the child are (the specific room within the facility or the location outside). Do not hang up the phone until told to do so by the EMS dispatcher.

Some early education programs have found it helpful to post a list of the items to tell the EMS dispatcher, including the actual street address and a description of how to get from the street into the facility. In an emergency, it is sometimes difficult to recall familiar information.

It is also important that on field trips and during outside activities, the caregiver or teacher has access to a telephone, knows how to contact the EMS system, and knows how to describe the current location of the ill or injured child.

Additional emergency preparations for the facility should include having basic first aid supplies throughout the facility. You also need a list of phone numbers for the poison center, local medical facilities, and up-to-date emergency contact information for each child's parent(s) or legal guardian(s). This information should be easily accessible.

Did You Know

Many EMS jurisdictions in the United States now have enhanced 9-1-1 service, with the ability to automatically identify the location of the emergency caller. However, mobile phone calls are not always identified by the enhanced 9-1-1 service. When calling 9-1-1 using a mobile phone, always provide your location to the EMS dispatcher.

First Aid Tip

These tips provide instant experience from masters of the trade.

Did You Know

This feature provides a better understanding of the topic presented.

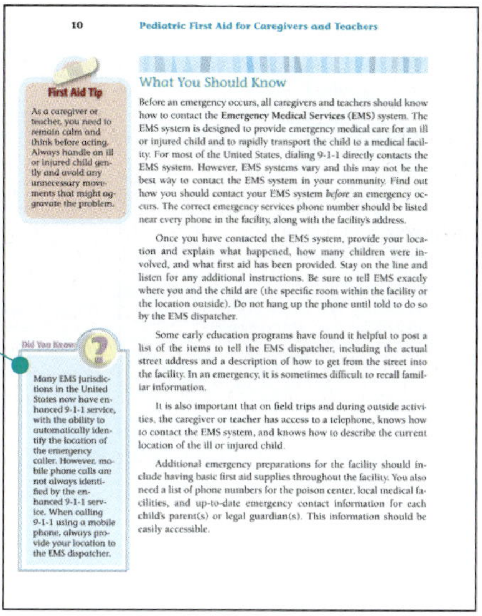

10 Pediatric First Aid for Caregivers and Teachers

First Aid Tip

As a caregiver or teacher, you need to remain calm and think before acting. Always handle an ill or injured child gently and avoid any unnecessary movements that might aggravate the problem.

What You Should Know

Before an emergency occurs, all caregivers and teachers should know how to contact the **Emergency Medical Services (EMS)** system. The EMS system is designed to provide emergency medical care for an ill or injured child and to rapidly transport the child to a medical facility. For most of the United States, dialing 9-1-1 directly contacts the EMS system. However, EMS systems vary and this may not be the best way to contact the EMS system in your community. Find out how you should contact your EMS system *before* an emergency occurs. The correct emergency services phone number should be listed near every phone in the facility, along with the facility's address.

Once you have contacted the EMS system, provide your location and explain what happened, how many children were involved, and what first aid has been provided. Stay on the line and listen for any additional instructions. Be sure to tell EMS exactly where you and the child are (the specific room within the facility or the location outside). Do not hang up the phone until told to do so by the EMS dispatcher.

Some early education programs have found it helpful to post a list of the items to tell the EMS dispatcher, including the actual street address and a description of how to get from the street into the facility. In an emergency, it is sometimes difficult to recall familiar information.

It is also important that on field trips and during outside activities, the caregiver or teacher has access to a telephone, knows how to contact the EMS system, and knows how to describe the current location of the ill or injured child.

Additional emergency preparations for the facility should include having basic first aid supplies throughout the facility. You also need a list of phone numbers for the poison center, local medical facilities, and up-to-date emergency contact information for each child's parent(s) or legal guardian(s). This information should be easily accessible.

Did You Know

Many EMS jurisdictions in the United States now have enhanced 9-1-1 service, with the ability to automatically identify the location of the emergency caller. However, mobile phone calls are not always identified by the enhanced 9-1-1 service. When calling 9-1-1 using a mobile phone, always provide your location to the EMS dispatcher.

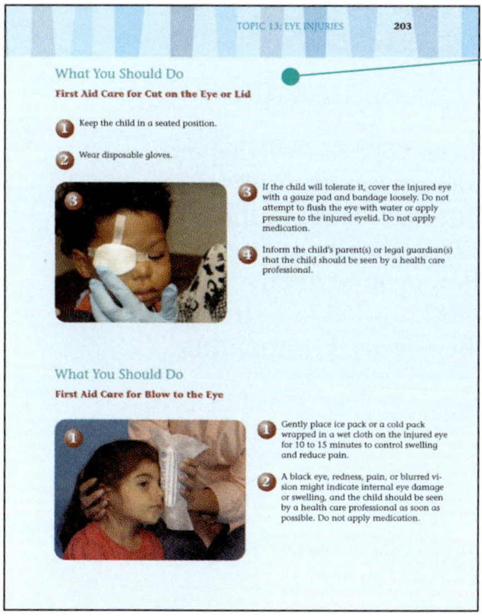

TOPIC 13: EYE INJURIES 203

What You Should Do

First Aid Care for Cut on the Eye or Lid

1. Keep the child in a seated position.
2. Wear disposable gloves.
3. If the child will tolerate it, cover the injured eye with a gauze pad and bandage loosely. Do not attempt to flush the eye with water or apply pressure to the injured eyelid. Do not apply medication.
4. Inform the child's parent(s) or legal guardian(s) that the child should be seen by a health care professional.

What You Should Do

First Aid Care for Blow to the Eye

1. Gently place ice pack or a cold pack wrapped in a wet cloth on the injured eye for 10 to 15 minutes to control swelling and reduce pain.
2. A black eye, redness, pain, or blurred vision might indicate internal eye damage or swelling, and the child should be seen by a health care professional as soon as possible. Do not apply medication.

First Aid Care

This feature provides short, step-by-step visual reviews of first aid procedures.

Resource Preview, continued

Algorithm

The algorithm is a flowchart designed to reinforce the decision-making process and appropriate first aid care.

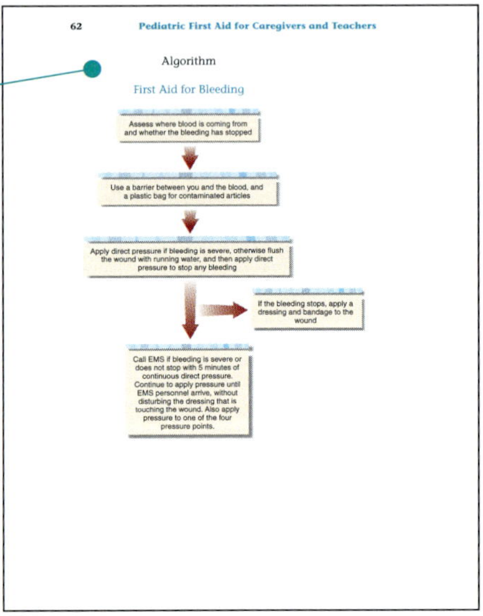
62 Pediatric First Aid for Caregivers and Teachers

Algorithm

First Aid for Bleeding

Assess where blood is coming from and whether the bleeding has stopped

Use a barrier between you and the blood, and a plastic bag for contaminated articles

Apply direct pressure if bleeding is severe, otherwise flush the wound with running water, and then apply direct pressure to stop any bleeding

If the bleeding stops, apply a dressing and bandage to the wound

Call EMS if bleeding is severe or does not stop with 5 minutes of continuous direct pressure. Continue to apply pressure until EMS personnel arrive, without disturbing the dressing that is touching the wound. Also apply pressure to one of the four pressure points.

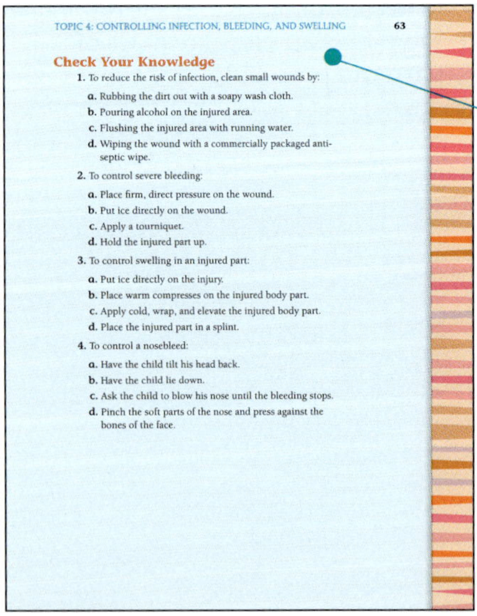
TOPIC 4: CONTROLLING INFECTION, BLEEDING, AND SWELLING 63

Check Your Knowledge

1. To reduce the risk of infection, clean small wounds by:
   a. Rubbing the dirt out with a soapy wash cloth.
   b. Pouring alcohol on the injured area.
   c. Flushing the injured area with running water.
   d. Wiping the wound with a commercially packaged antiseptic wipe.
2. To control severe bleeding:
   a. Place firm, direct pressure on the wound.
   b. Put ice directly on the wound.
   c. Apply a tourniquet.
   d. Hold the injured part up.
3. To control swelling in an injured part:
   a. Put ice directly on the injury.
   b. Place warm compresses on the injured body part.
   c. Apply cold, wrap, and elevate the injured body part.
   d. Place the injured part in a splint.
4. To control a nosebleed:
   a. Have the child tilt his head back.
   b. Have the child lie down.
   c. Ask the child to blow his nose until the bleeding stops.
   d. Pinch the soft parts of the nose and press against the bones of the face.

Check Your Knowledge

Check Your Knowledge provides an opportunity to test your knowledge of the first aid skills presented in the topic. It allows you to discover where your knowledge is strong and where it needs improving.

PedFACTs Resources

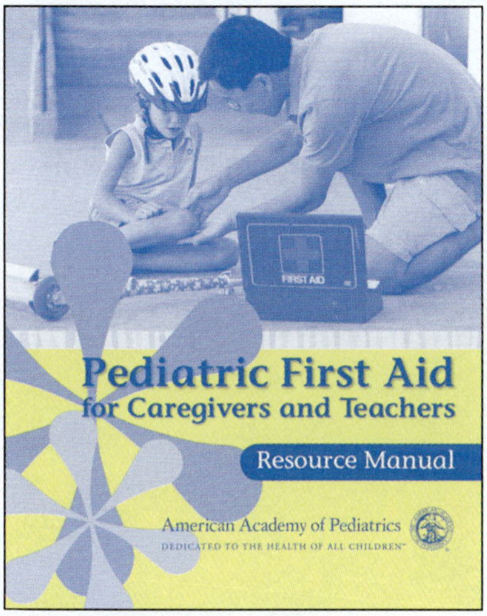

Resource Manual

ISBN: 0-7637-3640-6

An invaluable source of information, the Resource Manual contains:

- Helpful tips and guidelines for teaching a PedFACTs course
- Skill station strategies and activities
- Activities that will keep students engaged in group discussions
- Administrative information and forms

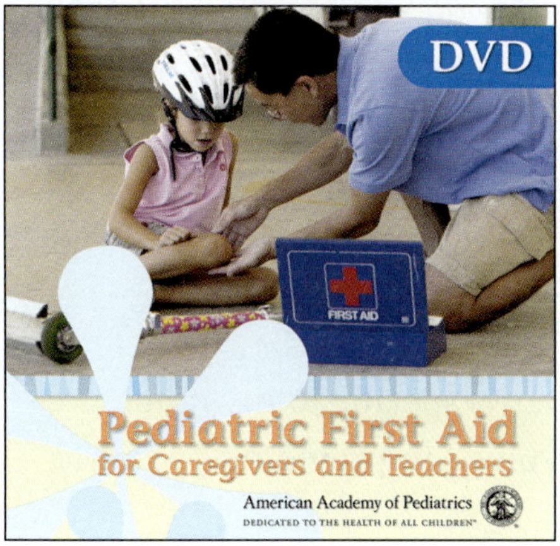

Video or DVD

ISBN: 0-7637-3643-0, DVD
ISBN: 0-7637-3642-2, VHS

Containing real-life footage, this video will captivate students and show them how to perform important skills and procedures.

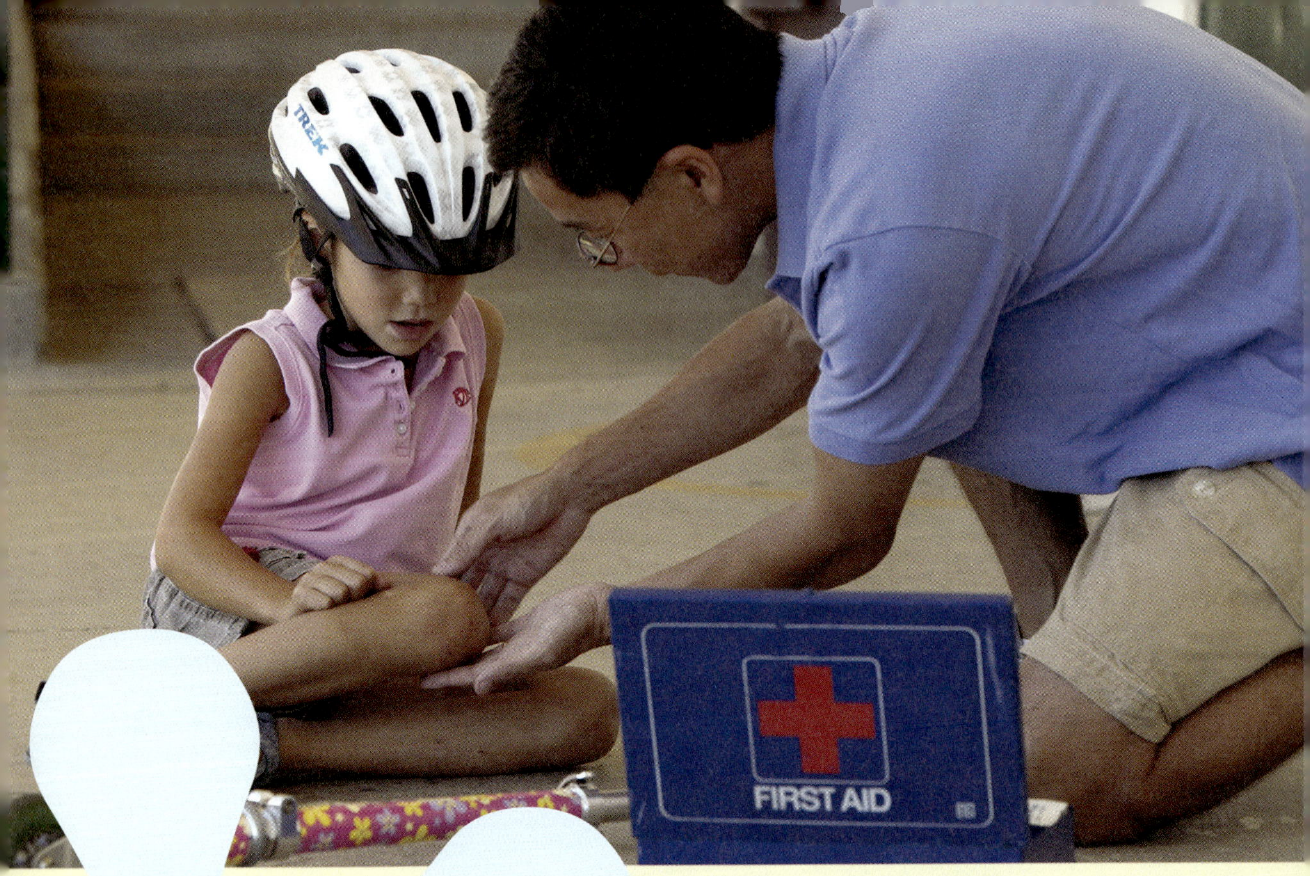

Learning Objectives

The participant will be able to:

- Define pediatric first aid.
- Identify Good Samaritan Laws specific to his state.
- Identify the eight steps involved in providing pediatric first aid.

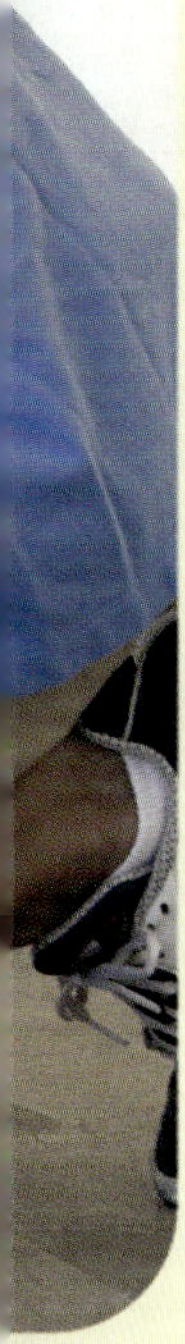

Topic 1 What is Pediatric First Aid?

What is Pediatric First Aid?

Caregivers and teachers need to know what to do when a child is injured or becomes suddenly and severely ill (**Figure 1-1**). Caregivers can include parents, legal guardians, relatives, and other individuals who care for children. **First aid** is the immediate care given to a suddenly ill or injured child until a medical professional or a parent or legal guardian assumes responsibility for the medical care of the child. First aid is intended to keep the child's medical condition from becoming worse and does not take the place of proper medical treatment. After providing first aid to a child, consultation with the parent(s) or legal guardian(s) and

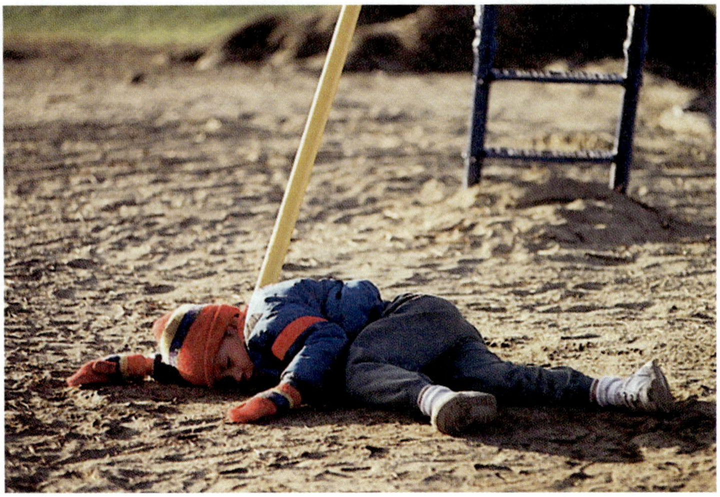

Figure 1-1

Caregivers and teachers need to know what to do when a child is injured or becomes suddenly and severely ill.

health professionals will determine what, if any, medical treatment is appropriate.

Most injuries that require first aid are not life-threatening. Usually, first aid involves simple, common sense procedures. However, first aid can sometimes mean the difference between life and death.

All caregivers and teachers should have pediatric first aid training (**Figure 1-2**). Many people use the term cardio-pulmonary resuscitation (CPR) to refer to all first aid skills. However, this is incorrect. CPR training focuses on what to do when the heart stops beating or when someone cannot breathe. It does not include what to do for all other types of injury or illness situations that might require first aid. For example, it does not teach caregivers and teachers what to do after a child falls and cuts his knee.

CPR is rarely required for children. For healthy children, the heart typically continues to beat unless the child stops breathing. If breathing stops due to choking, drowning, or a rare heart condition, the heart will eventually stop beating. For this reason, all caregivers and teachers should be trained in management of a blocked airway and rescue breathing. Caregivers and teachers who care for a child with a rare heart condition or who

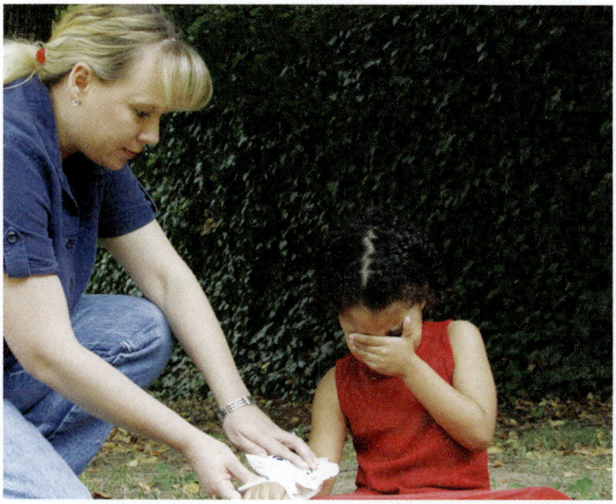

Figure 1-2

All caregivers and teachers should have pediatric first aid training.

supervise swimming or wading activities should be trained in CPR.

Caregivers and teachers are expected to provide the same quality of first aid that a layperson with first aid training could provide. Caregivers and teachers should also be able to obtain prompt help from the Emergency Medical Services (EMS) by dialing 9-1-1 or the local EMS phone number. If your facility is in a remote location or participates in activities in remote locations, then more advanced training may be required.

Caregivers and teachers have a duty to provide first aid to children in their care. Most states have a **Good Samaritan Law** that grants immunity from lawsuits to individuals providing first aid. Although laws vary from state to state, Good Samaritan immunity generally applies when the individual is acting during an emergency, acting in good faith, acting without compensation, and not guilty of any malicious misconduct or gross negligence. In addition, the law usually protects the individual from legal responsibility if he does what a reasonable person with the same amount of training would have done.

Did You Know ?

Situations for which CPR Training for Caregivers and Teachers is Required:

- Swimming and wading activities
- A child with a rare heart condition

> **First Aid Tip**
>
> The American Academy of Pediatrics and the American Public Health Association define pediatric first aid and CPR training required in out-of-home child care in Standard 1.026 through 1.028 of *Caring for Our Children: National Health and Safety Performance Standards: Guidelines for Out-of-Home Child Care,* 2nd edition, 2002. You can access this reference at http://nrc.uchsc.edu.

How Will I Learn Pediatric First Aid?

This is the participant manual for the American Academy of Pediatrics (AAP) *Pediatric First Aid for Caregivers and Teachers (PedFACTs)* course. It discusses illnesses and injuries that require first aid. The manual is intended as a reference for use during and after the course. It is organized so that topics include the following sections:

Learning Objectives: the expectations of what participants in the *PedFACTs* course will be able to do after successfully completing their training.

Introduction: an overview of the topic.

What You Should Know: more detailed background information about the topic.

What You Should Look For: the signs and symptoms that caregivers and teachers need to assess when caring for a child with a particular type of illness or injury.

What You Should Do: a reminder about the eight steps in pediatric first aid to follow in every situation that requires first aid, followed by topic-specific instructions for care.

Algorithm: step-by-step first aid instructions.

Check Your Knowledge: multiple choice questions at the end of the chapter to help you check your understanding of the topic.

You will see that key terms are in **bold type** to help you spot them easily. Also, each topic includes some additional information highlighted in boxes. These may include first aid tips, interesting information, a review of the essential items from the discussion, where to get more information, and illustrations.

As mentioned earlier, each topic will highlight the eight steps in pediatric first aid care. These steps are outlined below and will be discussed in more detail in *Finding Out What is Wrong* (see page 8).

The Eight Steps in Pediatric First Aid:

1 Survey the Scene

Take a brief moment to perform a scene survey to ensure that the scene is safe, to find out who is involved, and to determine what happened.

2 Hands-off ABCs

As you approach the child, perform the hands-off ABCs (Appearance, Breathing, and Circulation) to determine if EMS should be called. It should take 15 to 30 seconds or less.

3 Supervise

Immediately ensure that any other children near the scene are properly supervised.

4 Hands-on ABCDEs

Perform the hands-on ABCDEs (Appearance, Breathing, Circulation, Disability, and Everything else) to determine if EMS should be called and what first aid care is needed.

5 First Aid Care

Provide first aid care appropriate to the injury or illness.

6 Notify

As soon as possible, notify the child's parent(s) or legal guardian(s).

7 Debrief

As soon as possible, talk with the child who received first aid about any concerns he or she may have, and talk with other children who witnessed the injury and first aid procedures.

8 Document

Complete an incident report form.

Check Your Knowledge

1. Pediatric first aid is:

- **a.** Treatment to stop pain and to ensure healing after an injury or in the event of a life-threatening condition.
- **b.** The immediate care given to an injured or suddenly ill child.
- **c.** Required only if a child's parent(s) or legal guardian(s) cannot come quickly.
- **d.** Cardiopulmonary resuscitation.

2. State Good Samaritan Laws:

- **a.** Exempt someone who gives first aid from being sued for any care provided.
- **b.** Cover the same level of care for laypeople, doctors, and nurses who stop at the scene of an accident to offer pediatric first aid.
- **c.** Have different provisions from state to state, but generally protect against civil suit if the person does what would reasonably be expected.
- **d.** Require that someone who comes upon the scene of an accident must stop and offer to help.

3. Pediatric CPR training is needed:

- **a.** For all infant and toddler caregivers.
- **b.** For all caregivers and teachers.
- **c.** For caregivers and teachers who take care of children with seizures.
- **d.** For caregivers and teachers who supervise wading and swimming activities or care for a child with a rare heart condition.

4. Which of the items listed below is not one of the eight steps involved in pediatric first aid?

- **a.** Do a quick scene survey to be sure the scene is safe, to know who is involved, and what happened.
- **b.** Move the child to a comfortable place.
- **c.** Perform the hands-off ABCs as you approach the child, to see if EMS should be called immediately.
- **d.** Arrange for supervision of any other children in the group.

Terms

First Aid The immediate care given to an injured or suddenly ill child until a medical professional or parent(s) or legal guardian(s) assumes responsibility.

Good Samaritan Law A law passed in many states to protect individuals from liability when providing first aid.

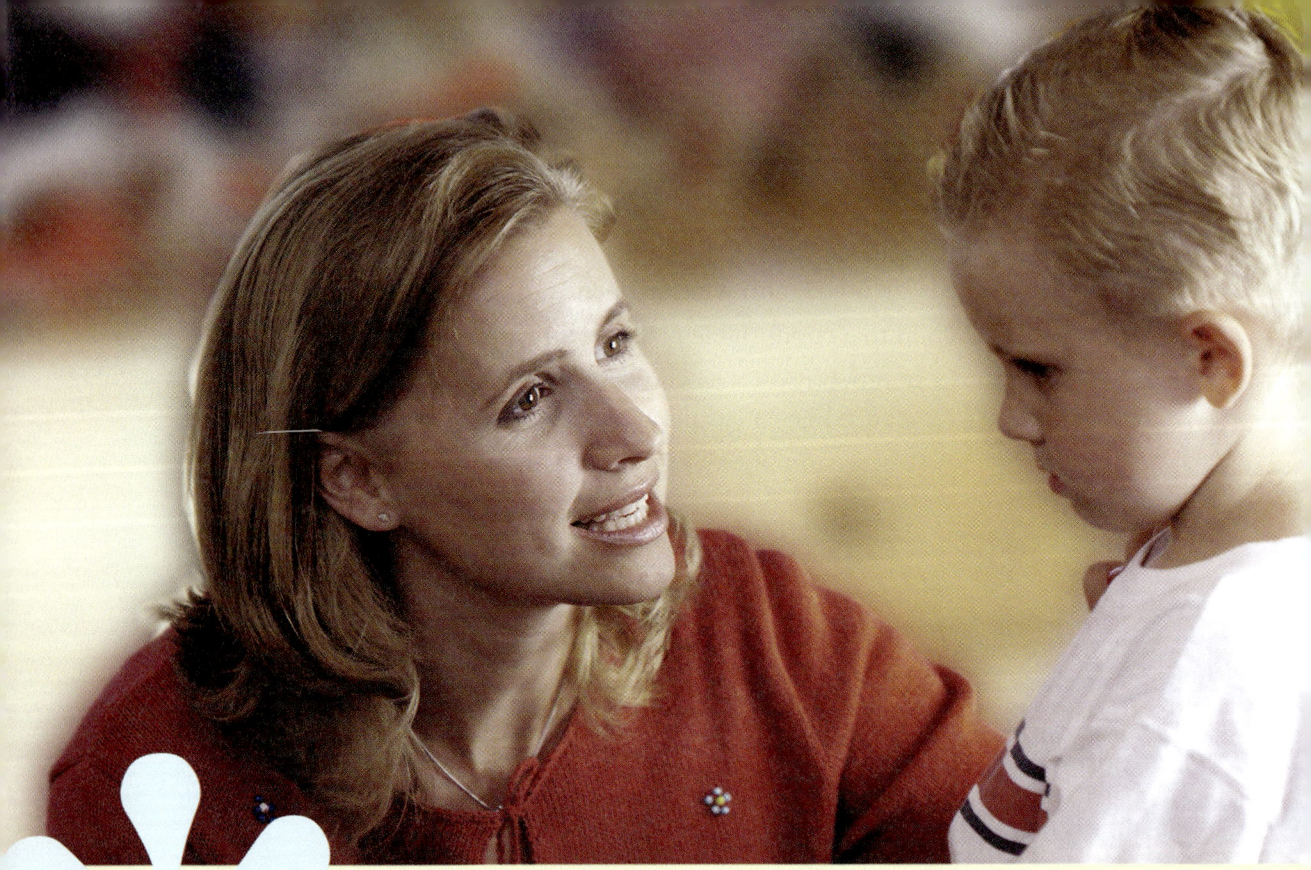

Learning Objectives

The participant will be able to:

- Describe how to perform a scene survey.
- Explain how to contact the EMS system.
- Describe how to perform the hands-off ABCs.
- Demonstrate how to perform the hands-on ABCDEs.
- Identify the eight steps in providing pediatric first aid from the scene survey to completion of the incident report.

Topic 2 Finding Out What is Wrong

Finding Out What is Wrong

Introduction

A 3-year-old boy falls from a playground slide and now lies on the ground crying. An 18-month-old girl gets into the cleaning supplies and now is vomiting. A 3-month-old infant has a fever of 103.6°F and looks pale. To find out what is wrong with each child, the caregiver or teacher must practice a calm and methodical approach. This approach will inspire the confidence of the injured child as well as any children witnessing the event.

What You Should Know

Before an emergency occurs, all caregivers and teachers should know how to contact the **Emergency Medical Services (EMS)** system. The EMS system is designed to provide emergency medical care for an ill or injured child and to rapidly transport the child to a medical facility. For most of the United States, dialing 9-1-1 directly contacts the EMS system. However, EMS systems vary and this may not be the best way to contact the EMS system in your community. Find out how you should contact your EMS system *before* an emergency occurs. The correct emergency services phone number should be listed near every phone in the facility, along with the facility's address.

First Aid Tip

As a caregiver or teacher, you need to remain calm and think before acting. Always handle an ill or injured child gently and avoid any unnecessary movements that might aggravate the problem.

Once you have contacted the EMS system, provide your location and explain what happened, how many children were involved, and what first aid has been provided. Stay on the line and listen for any additional instructions. Be sure to tell EMS exactly where you and the child are (the specific room within the facility or the location outside). Do not hang up the phone until told to do so by the EMS dispatcher.

Some early education programs have found it helpful to post a list of the items to tell the EMS dispatcher, including the actual street address and a description of how to get from the street into the facility. In an emergency, it is sometimes difficult to recall familiar information.

Did You Know

Many EMS jurisdictions in the United States now have enhanced 9-1-1 service, with the ability to automatically identify the location of the emergency caller. However, mobile phone calls are not always identified by the enhanced 9-1-1 service. When calling 9-1-1 using a mobile phone, always provide your location to the EMS dispatcher.

It is also important that on field trips and during outside activities, the caregiver or teacher has access to a telephone, knows how to contact the EMS system, and knows how to describe the current location of the ill or injured child.

Additional emergency preparations for the facility should include having basic first aid supplies throughout the facility. You also need a list of phone numbers for the poison center, local medical facilities, and up-to-date emergency contact information for each child's parent(s) or legal guardian(s). This information should be easily accessible.

Each caregiver and teacher should know about any child in her care who has a special health care need. Special health care needs include allergies to foods or medications, and specific conditions that may complicate first aid care, such as diabetes or asthma. Parent(s) or legal guardian(s) should be asked for permission to make the information about their child's special needs accessible, so that substitutes and volunteers can be made aware of any needs the child may have.

An **Emergency Information Form (EIF)** should be kept at home and on file at educational or recreational facilities for any child, including those with special health care needs. The EIF is a standardized form to inform EMS personnel who do not know about the child's medical problems and care. The child's parent(s) or legal guardian(s) and health care professional must fill out the form. The form includes the child's medical history, medications, allergies, equipment needs, common medical problems, and suggested initial treatments. A blank EIF is available at the American Academy of Pediatrics Web site. In the event of a medical emergency provide the EMS personnel with a copy of the child's EIF.

In addition to the EIF, each education program should have a special care plan for any child. The plan should highlight how to care for this child in case of an emergency involving the child or the group, such as the need to evacuate the facility. Developing a special care plan should involve input from the caregivers and teachers, the child's parent(s) or legal guardian(s), and the child's health care professional.

What You Should Look For

Some conditions warrant calling EMS, while others require prompt medical attention by a health care provider. If in doubt and concerned, you should always call EMS. While some specific conditions should signal a need for immediate medical care, your level of concern is also a good indicator. See Tables 2–1 and 2–2 for a list of conditions that require EMS and situations requiring medical attention.

Table 2–1 When to Call EMS

Call Emergency Medical Services (EMS) immediately for the following:

- Any time you believe a child needs immediate medical treatment
- Fever in association with an abnormal ABCs (appearance, breathing, or circulation)
- Multiple children affected by injury or serious illness at the same time
- A child is acting strangely, much less alert, or much more withdrawn
- Difficulty breathing, unable to speak
- Skin or lips that look blue, purple, or gray
- Rhythmic jerking of arms and legs and a loss of responsiveness (seizure)
- Unresponsive
- Decreasing responsiveness
- Any of the following after a head injury: decrease in level of alertness, confusion, headache, vomiting, irritability, difficulty walking
- Increasing or severe pain anywhere
- A cut or burn that is large, deep, and will not stop bleeding
- Vomiting blood
- A child with a severe stiff neck, headache, and fever
- A child who is significantly dehydrated: sunken eyes, not making tears or urinating, lethargic
- Suddenly-spreading purple or red rash
- A large volume of blood in the stools
- Hot or cold weather injuries (e.g., frostbite, heat exhaustion)

After you have called your local EMS, remember to call the child's parent(s) or legal guardian(s).

Table 2–2 Situations Requiring Medical Attention

Situations that do not necessarily require ambulance transport, but still need medical attention:

- Fever in any age child who looks more than mildly ill
- Fever of >100.5°F in a child less than 60 days (2 months) old
- Any age child who appears and is acting very ill
- Severe vomiting and/or diarrhea
- A serious cut that may require stitches (i.e., a wound that does not hold together by itself after cleaning)
- Any animal bites that puncture the skin
- Any venomous bites or stings with spreading local redness and swelling, or evidence of general illness
- Any medical condition specifically outlined in a child's care plan requiring parental notification

What You Should Do

The Eight Steps in Pediatric First Aid:

1 Survey the Scene

Take a brief moment to perform a scene survey to ensure that the scene is safe, to find out who is involved, and to determine what happened.

2 Hands-off ABCs

As you approach the child, perform the hands-off ABCs (Appearance, Breathing, and Circulation) to determine if EMS should be called. It should take 15 to 30 seconds or less.

3 Supervise

Immediately ensure that any other children near the scene are properly supervised.

4 Hands-on ABCDEs

Perform the hands-on ABCDEs (Appearance, Breathing, Circulation, Disability, and Everything else) to determine if EMS should be called and what first aid care is needed.

5 First Aid Care

Provide first aid care appropriate to the injury or illness.

6 Notify

As soon as possible, notify the child's parent(s) or legal guardian(s).

7 Debrief

As soon as possible, talk with the child who received first aid about any concerns he or she may have, and talk with other children who witnessed the injury and first aid procedures.

8 Document

Complete an incident report form.

Finding Out What is Wrong

1 Survey the Scene

Begin by taking a quick look at the area surrounding the child. Is the scene safe? Who is involved? What happened? (Safety?-Who?-What?) This quick look should take no more than 15 to 30 seconds.

First, ensure the *safety* of everyone at the scene, including yourself. Look for hazards such as deep water, fire, falling objects, a live electrical wire, or a dangerous animal. Although it is important to quickly reach the child in distress, you must first make sure that the scene is safe. For example, in the case of a fire, you should not rush into a burning building. This is the duty of a properly trained and equipped firefighter. Also, by observing the scene, you may see that more than one child is hurt, although the less seriously injured child may be first to draw your attention by crying. Skipping this step may place more people at risk and delay effective first aid.

> **First Aid Tip**
>
> The scene survey involves three tasks:
> **SAFETY:** Is the scene safe?
> **WHO:** Who is involved?
> **WHAT:** What happened?

Second, find out *who is involved.* Who may also be ill or injured? Are all of the children present? Who needs supervision or comforting? Who can help provide supervision and care for any other children in the group? Are other first aid providers available to help or to contact the EMS system?

If the scene is not safe and the child must be moved, use the shoulder drag method (**Figure 2-1**). To use this method, place one of your hands on each shoulder, with your forearms along the sides of the head to brace the child's neck during the move. Slowly drag the child to the nearest safe location, while continuing to brace the head and neck. For the child not suspected of having a spinal injury, move the child to a safe place by using the cradle carry for infants or younger children, and the ankle drag for older children (**Figure 2-2A, B**).

For the child who may have fallen, you must always consider the possibility of a spinal cord injury. If you need to move a child to safety, but a spinal cord injury is a possibility, do not move the child's head and neck. This may cause further spinal cord damage. Encourage injured children not to move if anything hurts. Comforting the ill or injured child without moving her is the safest approach. However, do not forcefully hold a child still. If a child can move all her body parts without pain, there is no need to force the child to hold still.

Third, find out *what happened.* Identify the possible causes or circumstances of the illness or injury. Did the child fall, and if so, from what height? Did the toddler choke on a missing part of a toy? Why is that stray dog near a bleeding child? Did two children run into each other? After completing the three-part scene survey, you will be able to provide safe and effective first aid.

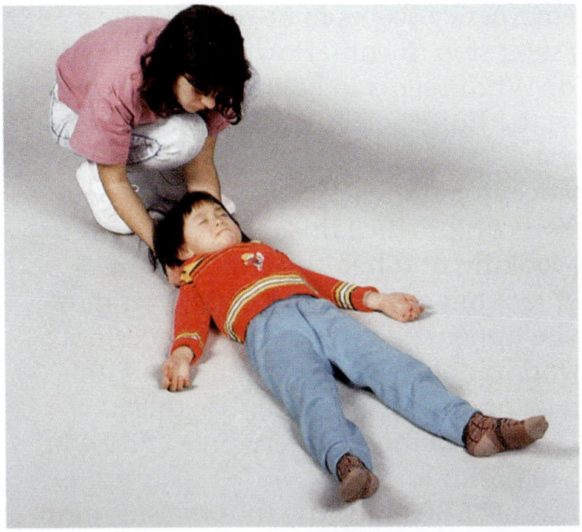

Figure 2-1

Shoulder drag.

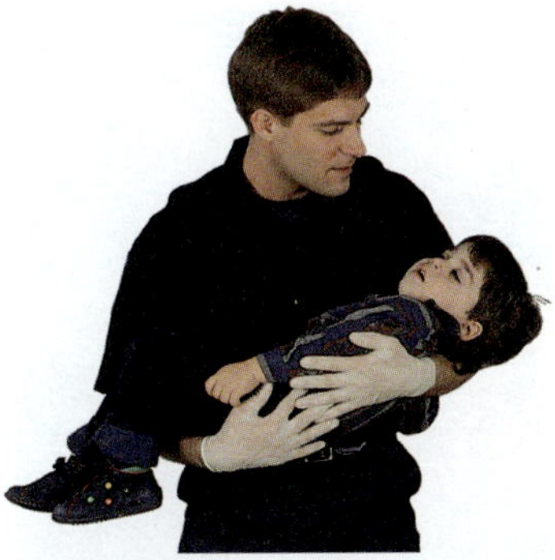

Figure 2-2A

Cradle carry.

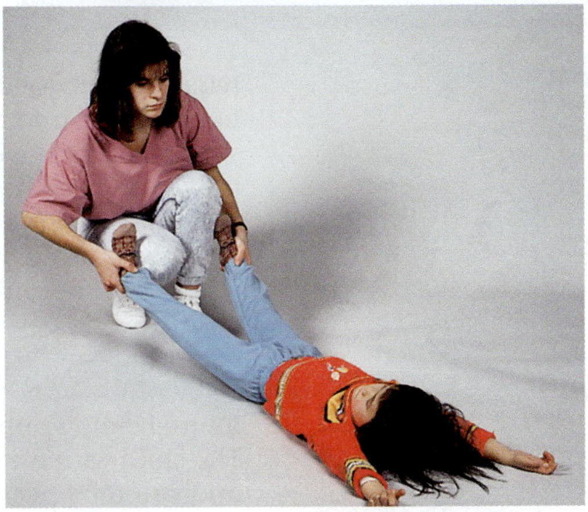

Figure 2-2B

Ankle drag.

2 Hands-off ABCs

Immediately following the scene survey, perform a check of the child called the **hands-off ABCs: A**ppearance, work of **B**reathing, and **C**irculation (based on skin color) to see if EMS should be called. The hands-off ABCs are done while you are approaching the ill or injured child, and before you begin care. This is your first chance to look at and listen to the ill or injured child. The hands-off check of the ABCs should take no more than 15 to 30 seconds.

The idea of looking and listening without touching the child who is ill or injured may seem counter to your natural desire to immediately begin to touch and do something for the ill or injured child. However, skipping this step may lead to an incorrect evaluation and management of the child's problem. Use the information from the hands-off ABCs to determine how

First Aid Tip

Hands-off ABCs
Appearance
Breathing (work of breathing)
Circulation (based on skin color)

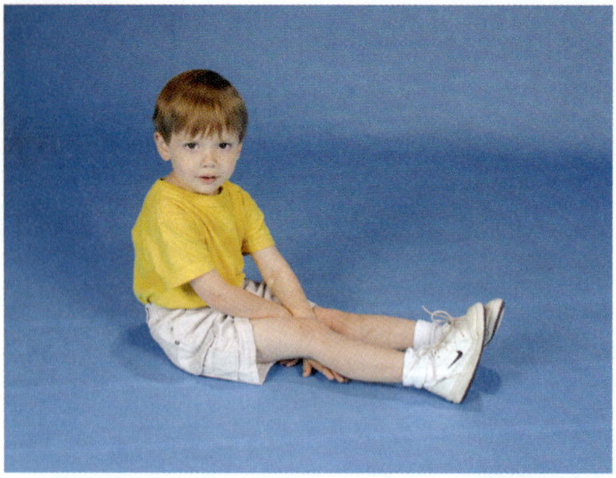

Figure 2-3

Appearance.

serious the emergency seems to be and the most appropriate next step in care. How badly is this child injured? What seems to be the child's main problem? Use the hands-off ABCs to decide first, and then act.

With practice, the hands-off ABCs can become automatic. You can practice this look and listen assessment by looking at a healthy child. For instance, when looking at a healthy child, you may notice that she appears active and alert, does not seem to be working harder than usual to breathe, and her skin color appears normal. Use this as a comparison when looking at a very pale child who is struggling to breathe.

If the hands-off ABCs indicate that the situation requires EMS, then ask someone else to call EMS if possible. If this is not possible, and the situation involves a breathing emergency, you should follow the instructions outlined in *Difficulty Breathing.* Provide the EMS dispatcher with the appropriate information and stay on the line until the EMS dispatcher says it is okay to hang up.

Be calm while you look at and listen to the child to determine the urgency of the child's problem. Remember, the purpose of the hands-off ABCs is to determine whether to call EMS immediately or to begin providing care.

'A' of the hands-off ABCs is for *Appearance* (**Figure 2-3**). The ill or injured child's appearance is the first and most important observation. The child with an abnormal appearance probably needs **urgent care**, and you may need to call EMS. Life-threatening situations always require calling the EMS.

First Aid Tip

Hands-off **'A'**:
Appearance
Alertness
Movement
Eye Contact

Appearance reflects how well the brain is functioning. How the infant or child interacts with her surroundings is an essential clue. Look at the ill or injured child's alertness, movement, and eye contact. Is the child active with good strength and normal movement, or limp and not moving? Note whether the child seems to respond to someone coming to help when you or another caregiver or teacher approach her. Does the child make eye contact with you, or does she stare off at nothing in particular?

'B' is for *Breathing.* The child who is working harder to breathe than would be normal for the situation probably needs urgent care, and you need to call EMS. Hands-off evaluation of breathing includes listening for abnormal sounds, looking for an abnormal breathing position, and looking for signs of increased effort.

First Aid Tip

Hands-off **'B'**:
Breathing
Abnormal Sounds or Position
Nasal Flaring

Is the child making snoring, grunting, wheezing, or gurgling noises with each breath? Is the child's cry or voice weak, hoarse, or muffled? Can the older child only speak a few words at a time? Does the child appear anxious or frightened because of difficulty breathing? Is the child choking?

The child with abnormal breathing often will be more comfortable in an upright position, and may be uncomfortable lying down. A child who is sitting in a **sniffing position**, with her head up and tilted forward, or who is sitting upright and leaning forward with abnormally deep breaths, may be experiencing difficulty breathing. **Nasal flaring,** or flaring of the nostrils is also an indication that the child is having difficulty breathing.

'C' is for *Circulation.* In the hands-off observation, you should note whether the child's skin color looks unusual. Unusual skin color for the situation suggests a problem with circulation. It should be considered abnormal, and a sign that you should call EMS to assess the child.

Abnormally light or pale skin color, or blue color **(cyanosis)** may indicate a problem with circulation (**Figure 2-4**). When young infants are cold, you may notice a blotchy 'marble' appearance to their skin. This is called **mottling.** A cold infant also may have bluish color feet and hands. Although pale skin, mottling, and cyanosis (particularly of the hands and feet) may be normal in the infant exposed to cold, it should improve as the infant is warmed up. It is abnormal for a warm child to have these signs. A child whose skin is unusually pink may be overheated or have a rash.

First Aid Tip

Hands-off **'C':**
Circulation
Light or pale skin
Cyanosis (bluish skin color)
Mottling (blotchy, marble appearance to skin)
Unusually pink skin

3 Supervise

If you are caring for more than one child, you need to arrange for supervision of any other children in the group before you can focus your attention on caring for the ill or injured child. The other children must stay safe. If other caregivers or teachers are available, ask one of them to take care of the other children, removing them from the area if possible. This will limit the exposure of the other children to the details and involvement in the situation. If you are alone, ask the other children to move away. You might ask them to sit down in a circle. You can tell them you are taking care of the child and you need their help to make the child feel better. You can ask them to sing familiar songs, look at books, or perform any other safe activity that requires minimal involvement from you.

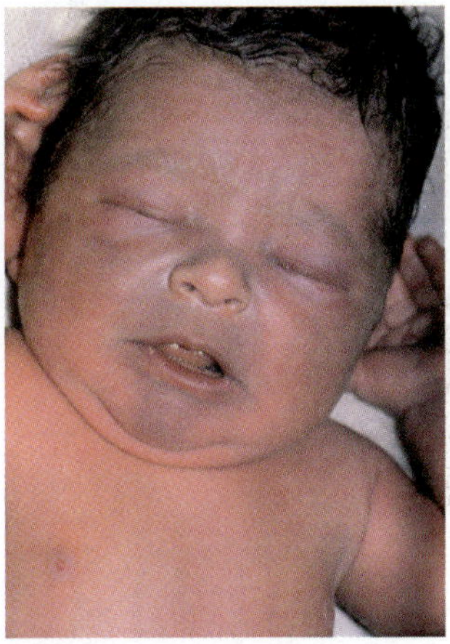

Figure 2-4

Cyanosis.

4 Hands-on ABCDEs

If the hands-off ABCs identify a potentially life-threatening illness or injury, or one that places the child at risk for permanent harm, make sure that you or another adult call EMS immediately. For the child who appears to have an illness or injury that does not require urgent care, you can begin to evaluate and manage the problem with first aid. The hands-on ABCDEs will guide you.

The **hands-on ABCDEs** are a closer look at the ABCs from the hands-off part of the evaluation, adding a 'D' (Disability) to look at how well the child can move on her own, and 'E' (Everything else) to check the child from head-to-toe for any ad-

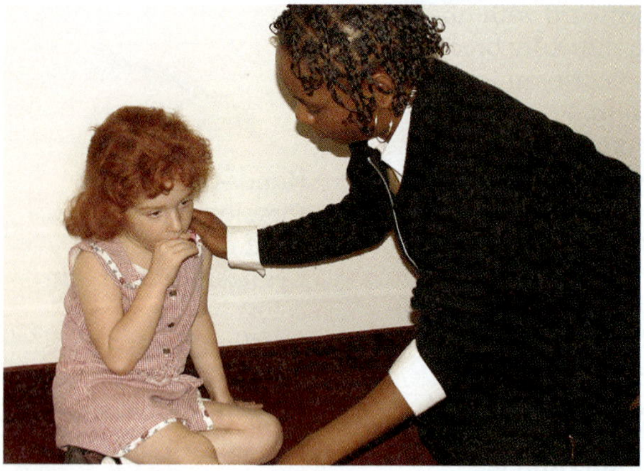

Figure 2-5

Hands-on ABCDEs.

ditional problems. The ABCDEs is a continuation of your initial assessment, once you reach the child, are able to touch the child, and examine the child's response. If at any time during the ABCDEs you discover that the child needs urgent care, you should call EMS immediately.

In the hands-on ABCDEs, 'A' involves a more detailed check of *Appearance*. Does the child respond to gentle touching and stimulation? Is the child's behavior normal under these circumstances? Does the child awaken and respond in a normal fashion? The infant or child with an abnormal appearance to hands-on ABCDEs may require urgent care by EMS.

During the hands-on ABCDEs, 'B' is for a more detailed check of *Breathing*. If, in the hands-off ABCs, the child is showing difficulty breathing, EMS should be contacted. If urgent care is not needed, the caregiver needs to continue to look for further signs of breathing difficulties. Continue to check for abnormal positioning or any changes in breathing patterns, and listen for any abnormal sounds while the child is breathing. If the child is not breathing see Topic 3, Difficulty Breathing.

'C' of the ABCDEs is for *Circulation*, a hands-on aspect to observations of skin color. Gently warm the infant or child who has been exposed to cold by adding layers of clothing or a blanket, and then note whether any abnormal coloring of the hands or feet improves. When there is bleeding, continue to monitor circulation while providing first aid. Mottling (blotchy, marble-like appearance to the skin) or cyanosis (blue color to the skin) requires urgent care from EMS. Other signs of circulation include breathing, coughing, and movement. If these do not exist, call EMS, and if trained, perform CPR.

'D' stands for *Disability* in the hands-on ABCDEs, which includes observing how well the ill or injured child can move. Does the child sit up, stand up, and move all body parts normally? Does the child squeeze your hand, wiggle her fingers and toes, and move her feet, hands, head, and trunk without stopping because of pain (**Figure 2-5**)? Do not move any body part that the child does not want moved, but gently touch the child to feel if the movements seem normal.

Finally, the hands-on ABCDEs should include 'E' for *Everything else*. Look the child over from head-to-toe. If the ill or injured child can talk, ask if anything hurts, and have the child point to where it hurts. You may need to lift up clothing to look at and gently touch the injured body parts. Does the child with a fever now have a rash? Does the child have reddened or blistered skin from the spilled hot water?

5 First Aid Care

This step is unique to each injury and illness. Your hands-off and hands-on assessments will determine what first aid care you should give to the ill or injured child. The recommended first aid care steps for the various injuries are identified in this text within the various topics.

6 Notify

This step is essential when the person providing first aid is not a parent or legal guardian of the child. Even when EMS medical attention is not required, you should notify the parent(s) or legal guardian(s) about the incident as soon as possible. Sometimes, another person can do this while you care for the child. Use your emergency contact information to locate the parent(s) or legal guardian(s). While the caregiver or teacher may not think the child needs care from a health care professional, the parent(s) or legal guardian(s) should have the opportunity to evaluate the situation and decide what to do.

Be calm when notifying the parent(s) or legal guardian(s). Give the facts about what happened to the child. If another child was involved in the event, do not reveal that child's identity. If EMS has been called, let the parent(s) or guardian(s) know where EMS will be taking the child so that they can go to the emergency facility to join the child as soon as possible. Tell the parent(s) or legal guardian(s) about the first aid that the child received, who provided first aid, and who is currently with the child.

7 Debrief

After you attend to the needs of the ill or injured child, and the proper individuals have been informed, you need to comfort and address the concerns of the child who received first aid and other children who witnessed the incident and first aid activities. Those who know the children well are best suited to handle this step. The type of comforting and explanation should be developmentally appropriate, and adapted to the temperament and response of the children in the group.

For infants and young toddlers, the approach might involve using a soothing and reassuring tone of voice. You can use a few gently spoken phrases such as "Johnny got hurt. We are making him feel better." Resuming routines as soon as possible helps.

For older children, a caregiver or teacher can ask the children what they think happened. Listen to what they say, affirm what is correct, and gently correct their misperceptions. Keep explanations simple and truthful. Minimize sharing graphic details that the children do not bring up themselves. It's a good idea to provide opportunities for children to work through the experience as long as they seem interested in it.

First Aid Tip

If a prescription medication was provided to a child in the child care setting, then an entry should be made in the report discussing the details of the administration of the medication, including the child's symptoms, the time the medication was administered, how much medication was given, who administered the medication, and the outcome of the use of the medications. This information should be shared with the child's parent(s) or legal guardian(s).

Some helpful activities are dramatic play, drawing, storytelling by the children, a non-emergency visit from an ambulance company crew, and reading books that relate to the experience. Although an emergency is stressful, the crisis provides an opportunity for children to learn about emergencies and how to cope with them.

Since the children who receive or witness first aid in an out-of-home setting may need more comforting at home, be sure to let parent(s) or legal guardian(s) know that there was an emergency during the day. Do not share confidential details, but make the parent(s) or legal guardian(s) aware of what their child may have seen or heard that was unusual for them. Some children may want to talk about the experience at home. Some may show signs or symptoms of having their day's routines upset, such as difficulty sleeping. Others may bring up what they have observed at some other time when the memory of the emergency is triggered by another event. Parent(s) or legal guardian(s) will appreciate being able to understand their children's reactions.

Even seasoned health professionals feel stress when a child has a medical emergency. Talking about what happened and about the feelings related to it can help cope with stress. Plan time to talk.

8 Document

In an education or child care setting, you need to fill out an incident report for any first aid activities. The caregiver or teacher should carefully document the details of the illness or injury, the first aid provided, the time and details of the call for medical help, the call to the parent(s) or legal guardian(s), and the outcome for the child of the event. Careful documentation is important. Some details are best recorded right away; others may require a day or two before you have the information you need to finish the report. Having a few days to reflect on what happened can be helpful. What you record should always be accurate and objective.

Incident reports help programs for education and child care, parents, legal guardians, insurance companies, and attorneys document what happened. Administrators who review the forms may help staff think about ways to prevent the situation from happening again. Education programs find it helpful to keep a file of incident reports that they routinely review every 3 to 6 months. A systematic review can identify patterns that suggest a hazardous condition that may not be apparent after a single event.

Algorithm

Finding Out What is Wrong

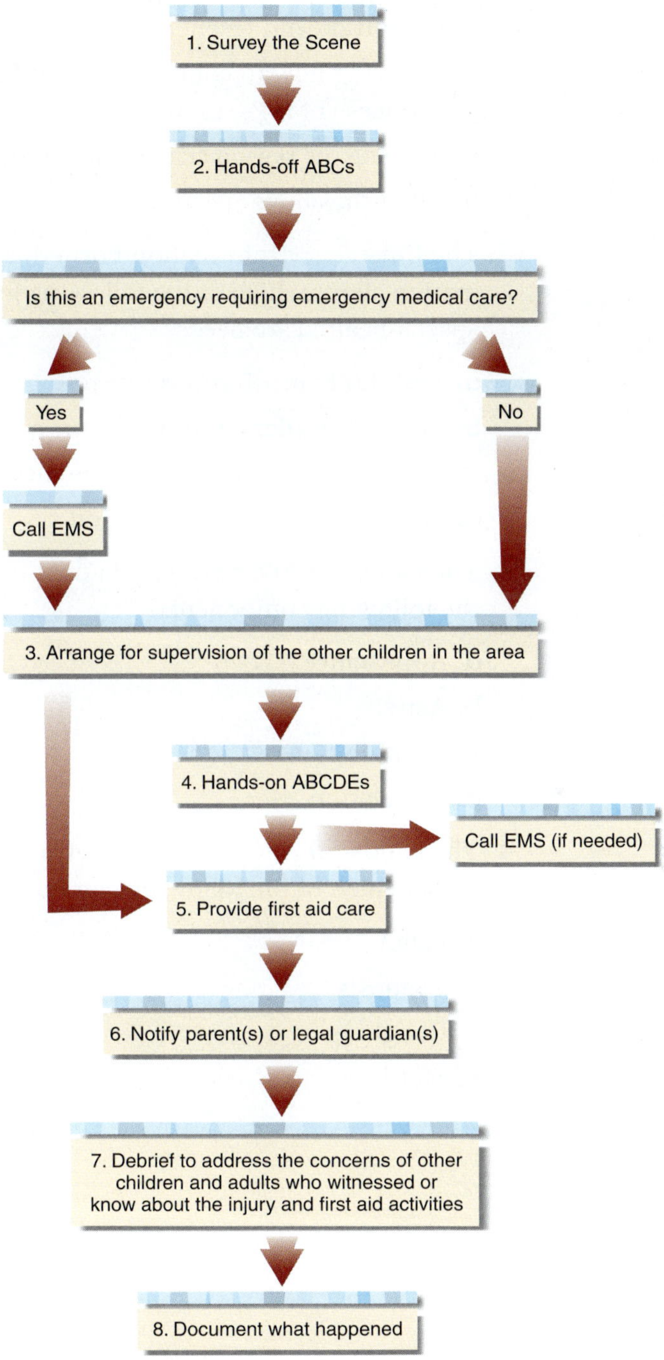

Check Your Knowledge

1. Which of the following is a part of preparing for an emergency?

   a. Caregivers and teachers completing a first aid course

   b. Knowing how to contact the local Emergency Medical Services (EMS) system

   c. Keeping the poison center number by the phones

   d. All of the above

2. The Emergency Information Form does *not* provide information about which of the following for the child with special health care needs?

   a. The child's medications

   b. The child's allergies to medications

   c. Common medical emergencies the child may have

   d. Medical insurance information

3. The hands-off ABCs evaluation does *not* include which of the following components?

   a. Appearance

   b. Activity

   c. Breathing

   d. Circulation

4. The hands-off ABCs evaluation of circulation does not include which of the following components?

   a. Pallor

   b. Cyanosis

   c. Coughing

   e. Mottling

Terms

Cyanosis	Slightly bluish discoloration of the skin.
Emergency Information Form (EIF)	A standardized form for use across the United States that is filled out by the child's parent(s) or legal guardian(s) and the health care professional for a child with special health care needs.
Emergency Medical Services (EMS)	A system that represents the combined efforts of several professionals and agencies to provide emergency medical care.
Hands-off ABCs	The "across the room" assessment performed by someone who is approaching the ill or injured child who is in need of first aid. It includes assessment of appearance, work of breathing, and circulation (based on skin color).
Hands-on ABCDEs	The assessment done after the hands-off ABCs. It includes a more detailed assessment of appearance, breathing, circulation, disability, and everything else.
Mottling	A blotchy marble-like appearance to the skin.
Nasal flaring	When infants and young children are working hard to breathe, they often will open or flare their nasal passages with each attempt to breathe air in.
Sniffing position	When the child sits with head slightly elevated and is leaning forward as if she were sniffing a flower.
Urgent care	Care provided by EMS or another medical professional.

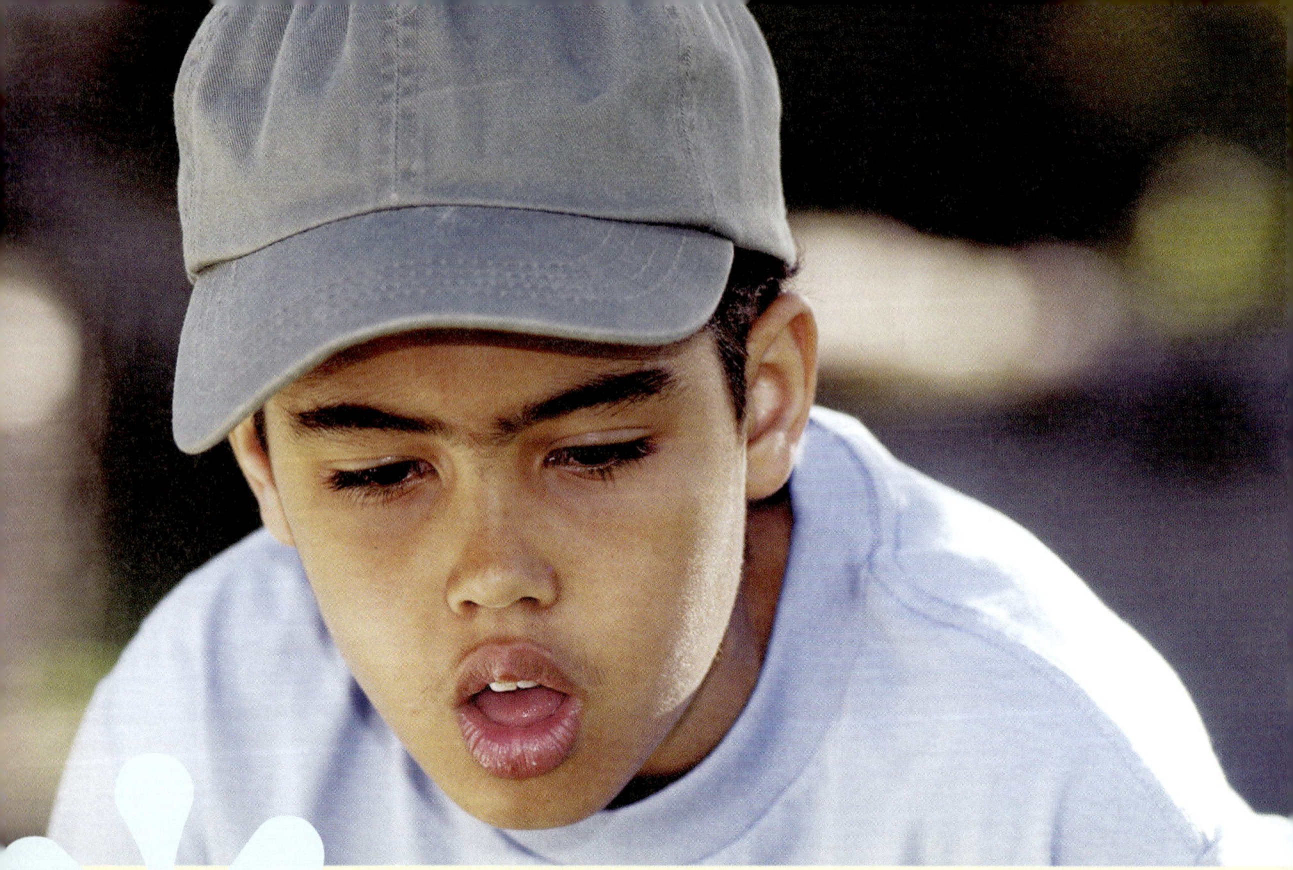

Learning Objectives

The participant will be able to:

- Recognize an infant or child who is unresponsive and call EMS.
- Recognize an infant who is having difficulty breathing and determine if first aid for a blocked airway is needed.
- Recognize a child who is having difficulty breathing and determine if rescue breathing is needed.
- Demonstrate the management of a blocked airway on an infant manikin.
- Demonstrate the management of a blocked airway on a child manikin.
- Demonstrate rescue breathing.

Topic 3

Difficulty Breathing

Difficulty Breathing

Introduction

The body needs oxygen to live. Oxygen enters the body through the lungs, where it passes into the blood. The heart circulates the oxygen-rich blood into every cell in the body, and the most demanding user of oxygen is the brain. The brain can survive for only a few minutes without oxygen before brain damage is likely to occur (**Figure 3-1**). This is why **respiratory arrest** (when breathing stops) and **cardiac arrest** (when the heart stops) are the most urgent life-threatening emergencies.

Figure 3-1

Brain damage occurs quickly if oxygen is not delivered.

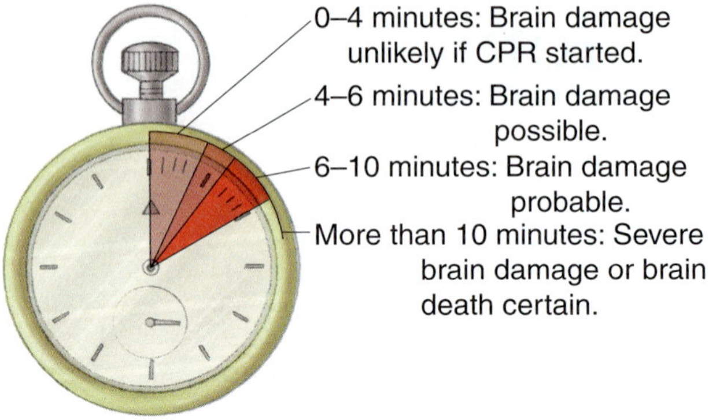

What You Should Know

Cardiac arrest rarely occurs in children. For most children, the heart is a healthy, strong muscle that pumps blood through the body. When a child's heart stops beating, it is seldom caused by a problem within the heart. Rather, it is usually the result of an injury that first caused the child to be unable to breathe. The most common causes for breathing problems in infants and young children are respiratory infection, choking, and drowning. Asthma and allergic reactions may also cause swelling in the airway that can lead to difficulty breathing (**Figure 3-2**).

Figure 3-2

The respiratory system.

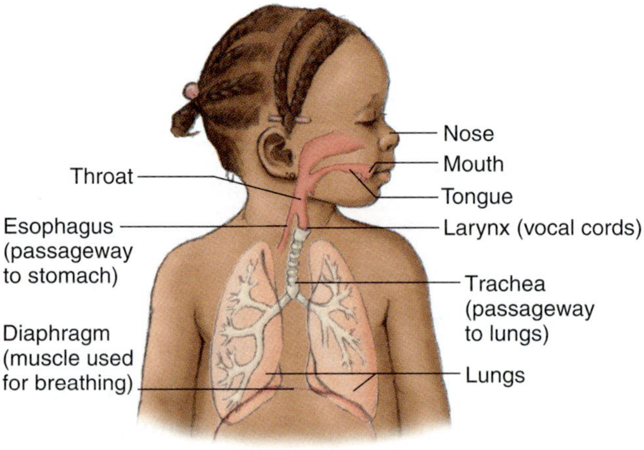

Did You Know?

Except for children with cardiac problems, or in cases of drowning, a child's heart typically does not stop beating unless the child first stops breathing. Therefore, cardiopulmonary resuscitation (CPR) training is necessary for facilities that enroll children with conditions that may result in cardiac arrest or those programs that have higher risk activities such as swimming. All caregivers in early education and child care settings should learn how to manage a blocked airway and provide rescue breathing.

Quickly removing an object that is blocking the airway so that air can get into the lungs is called management of a blocked airway. Breathing cannot occur if the airway is blocked. Getting air back into the lungs of a child who is not breathing is called **rescue breathing.** Management of a blocked airway and rescue breathing are the most important and critical skills that anyone who cares for children of any age can learn. A child may die unless management of a blocked airway and rescue breathing are started while waiting for EMS personnel to arrive.

What You Should Look For

Choking is a preventable, but common problem. A child may put a coin, button, or small toy in his mouth, or bite a latex balloon and take a breath, sucking the object into his airway. An object lodged in the airway can cause a partial (mild) or complete (severe) blockage. A completely blocked airway prevents oxygen from entering the lungs. An infant or child with a completely blocked airway will become unresponsive within minutes if the object is not removed. When a child has a completely blocked airway, he is generally unable to cry, speak, breathe, or cough. When you ask an older child who has a blocked airway, "Can you speak?" he is unable to respond verbally. An older child who is choking may instinctively reach and clutch his neck, to signal that he is choking. This motion is known as the **universal distress signal** for choking (**Figure 3-3**).

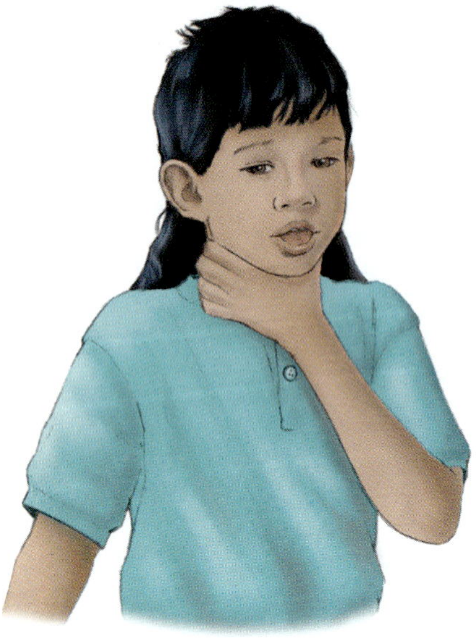

Figure 3-3

Universal distress signal.

An infant or child with a partially blocked airway continues to breathe, but will usually be coughing and anxious. Coughing is the body's way of removing what feels like a foreign object. This feeling occurs when there is swelling, irritation, or mucus anywhere in the airway. This is why people often cough when they have sinusitis or a runny nose. When there is an object in the airway, forceful coughing is more effective than anything anyone else can do to get the object to move up and out of the airway.

A child with difficulty breathing may also have respiratory distress. Respiratory distress most commonly occurs in children with asthma or wheezing. Wheezing can come on suddenly. A child who is known to have wheezing problems may have a prescription medicine that can help relieve wheezing. Caregivers and teachers should follow the instructions for using this medicine without delay.

Children with asthma or an airway infection who are working hard to breathe may tire and stop breathing. This requires EMS. The caregiver or teacher must provide rescue breathing while waiting for EMS personnel to arrive.

When a child has been submerged in water and is not breathing, this is called drowning. The nonbreathing child who has suffered a suffocation injury from submersion in water will need rescue breathing while EMS is en route.

The most important signs to recognize are those that show you that a child is working hard to breathe. You may see some of the signs of difficulty breathing:

- Drooling (unrelated to teething) occurs when a child is unable to swallow saliva either because of swelling in the back of his throat or because it is hard to swallow saliva while leaning forward and working hard to breathe.
- Head bobbing may occur when the child is working hard to breathe. The strong contraction of the neck muscles may move the head and pull up on the chest.

- **Nasal flaring** occurs when a child automatically opens or flares his nasal passages with each attempt to breathe air in, trying to get as much air in as possible (**Figure 3-4**).
- **Sniffing position** is the way a child lifts his head slightly and leans forward as if he is sniffing a flower while trying to get more air into his lungs.
- **Tripod position** is the way a child will lean forward with outstretched arms, usually placed on top of the knees to make the best use of respiratory muscles.
- **Wheezing** is the production of whistling sounds when the child breathes. This sound is a result of swelling or blockage of the small tubes (bronchials) in the lungs.

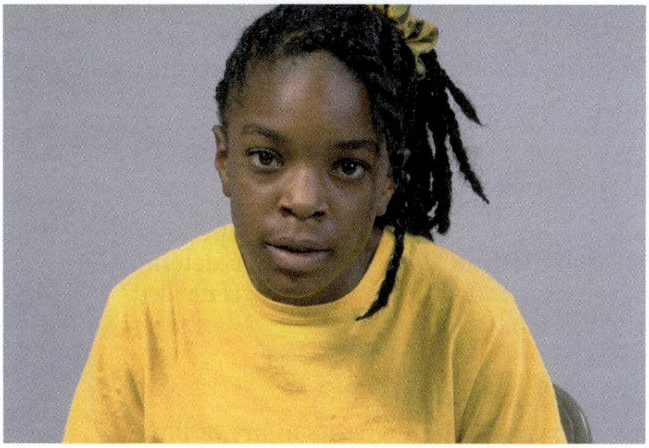

Figure 3-4

Nasal flaring.

What You Should Do

The Eight Steps in Pediatric First Aid:

1 Survey the Scene

Take a brief moment to perform a scene survey to ensure that the scene is safe, to find out who is involved, and to determine what happened.

2 Hands-off ABCs

As you approach the child, perform the hands-off ABCs (Appearance, Breathing, and Circulation) to determine if EMS should be called. It should take 15 to 30 seconds or less.

3 Supervise

Immediately ensure that any other children near the scene are properly supervised.

4 Hands-on ABCDEs

Perform the hands-on ABCDEs (Appearance, Breathing, Circulation, Disability, and Everything else) to determine if EMS should be called and what first aid care is needed.

5 First Aid Care

Provide first aid care appropriate to the injury or illness.

6 Notify

As soon as possible, notify the child's parent(s) or legal guardian(s).

7 Debrief

As soon as possible, talk with the child who received first aid about any concerns he or she may have, and talk with other children who witnessed the injury and first aid procedures.

8 Document

Complete an incident report form.

For any emergency situation, follow the eight steps for pediatric first aid. When you see that the child is having difficulty breathing, you must call EMS and provide first aid care for the breathing problem before you do anything else.

What You Should Do

First Aid for a Responsive Infant or Child with a Blocked Airway

Do not start management of a partially blocked airway (mild airway obstruction) if the infant or child can breathe, cry, speak, or cough. A good cough is more effective than anything you can do to clear the airway. If a child cannot breathe, cough, or make a normal voice sound and is still responsive, have someone call EMS as you begin first aid care. If you are alone, call EMS after providing 2 minutes of first aid care.

The technique for managing a blocked airway in a responsive infant (less than 1 year of age) consists of repeating a combination of 5 back slaps and 5 chests thrusts. To perform back slaps on an infant, turn the infant's head down on your forearm, with his feet up toward your shoulder. Place your hand around the infant's jaw and neck. The infant's head should be at a height lower than your trunk. Rest your arm against your thigh for support. Using the heel of your hand, give 5 quick, sharp back slaps between the infant's shoulder blades (**Figure 3-5**).

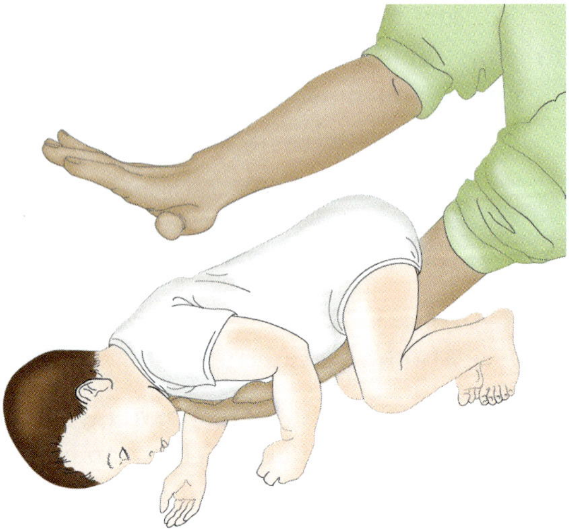

Figure 3-5

Using the heel of your hand, give 5 quick, sharp back slaps between the infant's shoulder blades.

Did You Know ?

Back slaps are used for responsive choking infants because the infant's chest is small and flexible. Giving back slaps with the infant's head down may cause enough chest movement that, in combination with gravity, may move the foreign object toward the mouth. If the object is moved a little, the infant may be able to cough the object out.

After doing 5 back slaps, give 5 chest thrusts. To perform chest thrusts on an infant, place your free hand on the back of the infant's head and neck, keeping the other hand that is supporting the head in place. Use both hands and forearms (one on the back and one on the front of the infant's body) to firmly hold the infant's body as you turn the infant over (**Figure 3-6**). Once turned onto his back, the infant should be resting on your arm, with your arm against your thigh. The infant's head should be lower than your trunk. Place two fingers on the infant's breastbone slightly below the nipple line. Avoid the bottom tip of the breastbone. Give 5 chest thrusts in rapid succession, pushing the breastbone down $\frac{1}{3}$ to $\frac{1}{2}$ the depth of the chest.

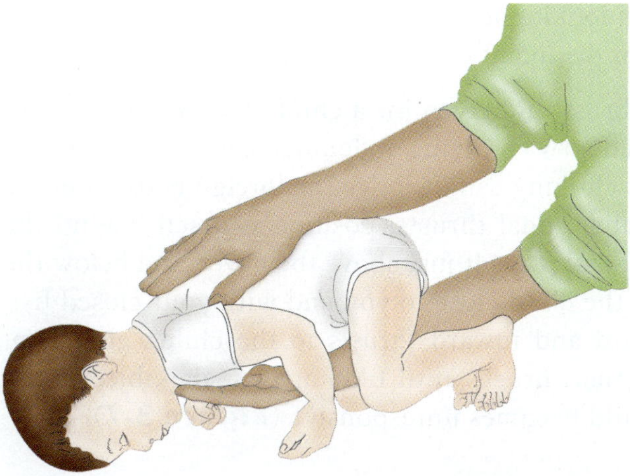

Figure 3-6

Use both hands and forearms (one on the back and one on the front of the infant's body) to firmly hold the infant's body as you turn the infant over.

Check inside the infant's mouth after you do the chest thrusts. If you see the foreign object, carefully remove it. Do not attempt a blind finger sweep to remove an object that you cannot see, since you might push it deeper. Continue alternating back slaps and

First Aid Tip

For a responsive infant who is choking:

1. Call EMS*
2. Give 5 back slaps
3. Give 5 chest thrusts
4. Check the mouth
5. Continue alternating 5 back slaps with 5 chest thrusts until EMS arrives, the foreign body is removed, or the infant becomes unresponsive

*If you are alone, provide 2 minutes of first aid and then call EMS.

chest thrusts, and looking for an object until EMS arrives, the object is removed, or the infant becomes unresponsive.

Abdominal thrusts are given for a child (1 to 8 years of age) who has a blocked airway. Giving abdominal thrusts to a responsive child who is choking can dislodge the foreign body from the airway. To give abdominal thrusts, position yourself behind the child. Make a fist and place it just above the navel, and below the breastbone. Pull the child close to you and with your closed fist, give quick upward and inward thrusts to the child's abdomen. Continue abdominal thrusts until EMS arrives, the object is removed, or the child becomes unresponsive (**Figure 3-7**).

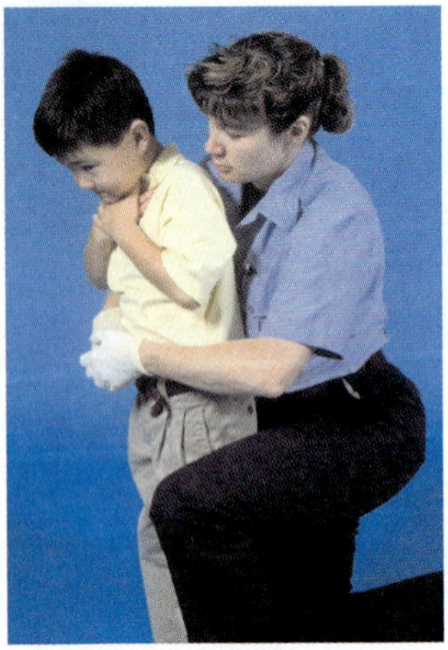

Figure 3-7

Continue abdominal thrusts until EMS arrives, the object is removed, or the child becomes unresponsive.

First Aid Tip

For a responsive child (1 to 8 years of age) who is choking:
- Call EMS*
- Give abdominal thrusts
- Continue until EMS arrives, the object is removed, or the child becomes unresponsive

*If you are alone, provide 2 minutes of first aid and then call EMS.

What You Should Do

First Aid for an Infant or Child Who is Unresponsive and Not Breathing

Rescue breathing is the technique to use when the infant or child is not breathing. If an infant or child is unresponsive and is not breathing or is choking and becomes unresponsive, you need to begin rescue breathing. The steps for rescue breathing include:

1. **Check for responsiveness:** The first step is to determine if you need to do rescue breathing. You do not use rescue breathing on a responsive infant or child. Gently tap the infant's or child's body and shout, "Are you okay?" (**Figure 3-8**).

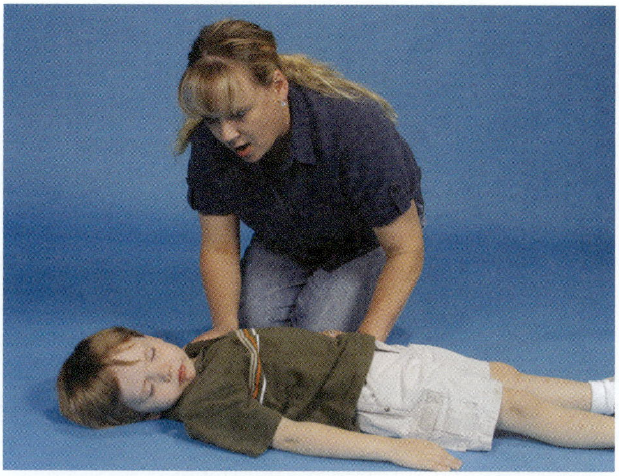

Figure 3-8

Check for responsiveness.

2. **Call EMS**: If the infant or child is unconscious/unresponsive, shout for help and ask someone to call 9-1-1 or the local emergency telephone number. If there is no one to help, perform 2 minutes of care before calling EMS (**Figure 3-9**).

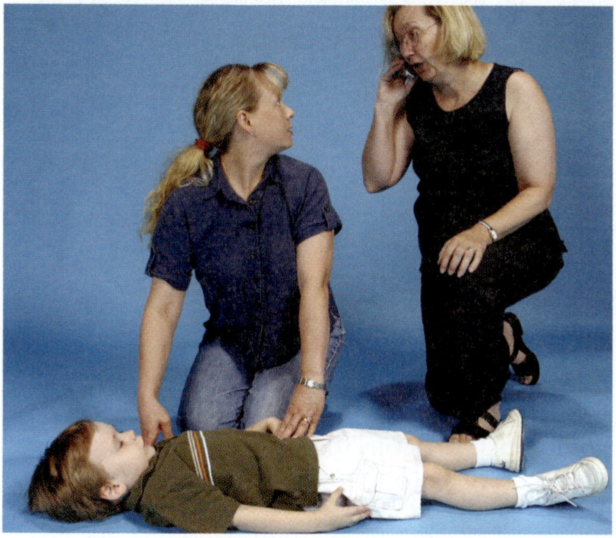

Figure 3-9

Call EMS.

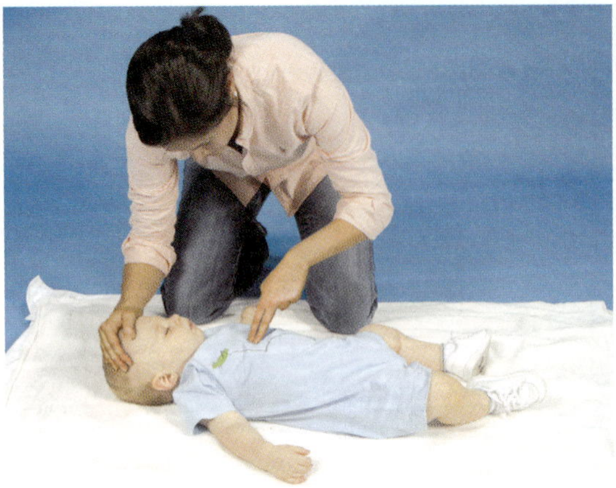

Figure 3-10A

Compress the chest of an infant 1⁄3 the depth of the chest, or about 4 cm (at least 1.5 inches).

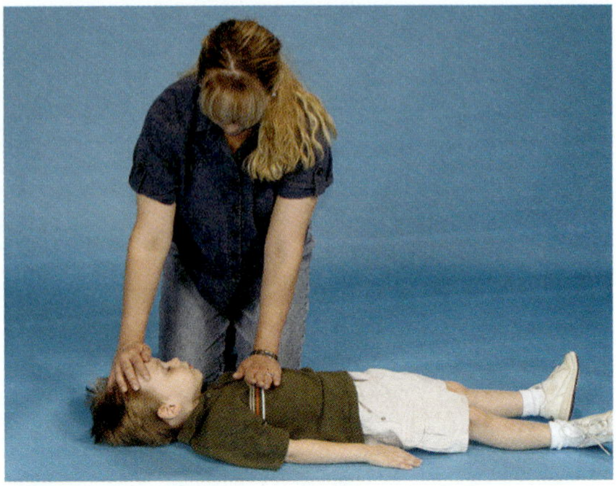

Figure 3-10B

Compress the chest of a child 1⁄3 the depth of the chest, or about 5 cm (at least 2 inches).

3. **Begin alternating 30 chest compressions and 2 rescue breaths**. Compress the chest of an infant 1⁄3 the depth of the chest, or about 4 cm (at least 1.5 inches) (**Figure 3-10A, B**). For a child, compress the chest 1⁄3 the depth of the chest, or about 5 cm (at least 2 inches).

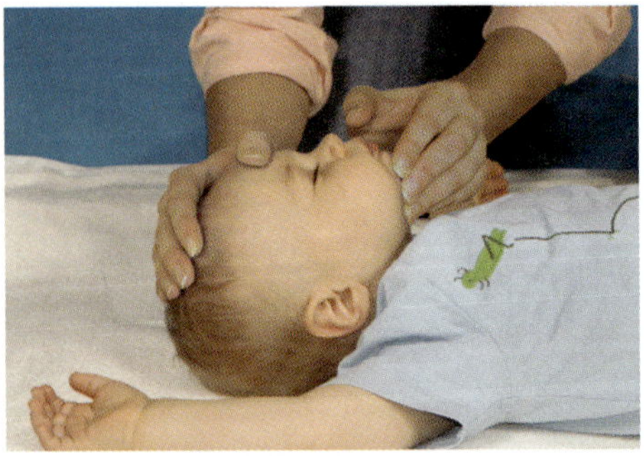

Figure 3-11

The head-tilt/chin-lift method.

4. **Open the airway:** Use the head-tilt/chin-lift method (**Figure 3-11**). To do this, place your hand on the infant's or child's forehead and tilt the head back slightly. Place the fingers of your other hand under the chin and lift gently; avoid pressing on the soft tissues under the jaw.
5. **Look in the mouth for an object:** Look for an object that you can remove easily. Do not perform a blind finger sweep of the mouth. Your attempts could push the object into the airway.
6. **Give rescue breaths.** If you do not see an object in the infant's or child's mouth and he does not start to breathe after opening the airway, give two breaths (1 second per breath), enough so that

you can see the chest rise and fall. The difference between the way you give rescue breaths for a child and for an infant is the way in which you seal your mouth over the airway to breathe air into the lungs. For the infant, you tilt the head back and seal your mouth over the infant's nose and mouth, and breathe into the nose and mouth (**Figure 3-12A**). For the child, you may have difficulty sealing your mouth around the child's mouth and nose (**Figure 3-12B**). Instead, pinch the child's nose, and then breathe into the child's mouth. Allow air to flow out of the chest after each breath. Each breath should take 1 second for air entry and about the same amount of time to allow for the air to flow out of the chest. If the chest does not rise and fall with the attempt to give the first breath, reposition the head and chin to open the airway and attempt to give another breath. Continue providing rescue breaths and chest compressions until the infant or child begins breathing or EMS arrives.

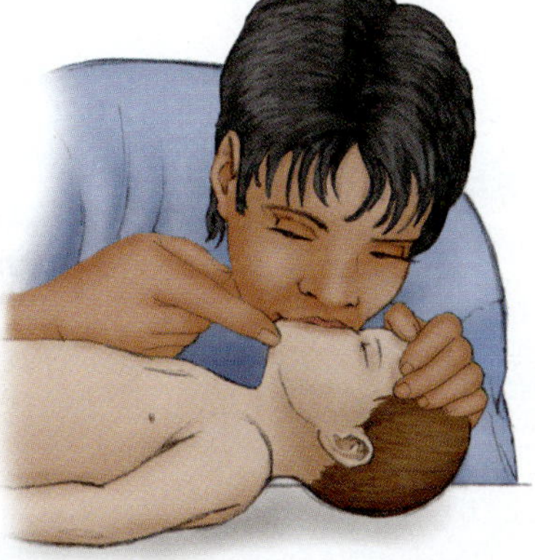

Figure 3-12A

For the infant, you tilt the head back and seal your mouth over the infant's nose and mouth, and breathe into the nose and mouth.

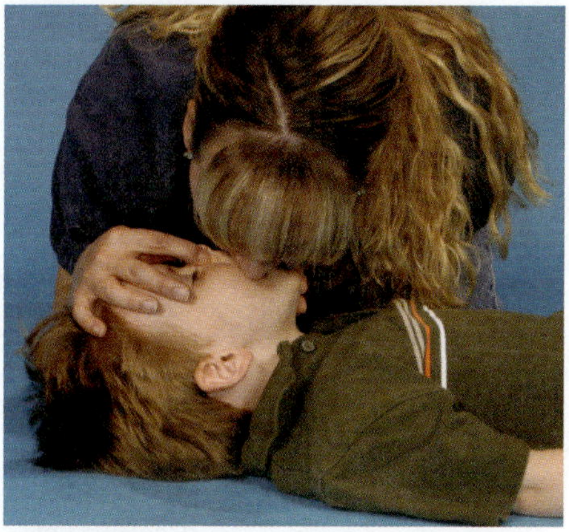

Figure 3-12B

For the child, you may have difficulty sealing your mouth around the child's mouth and nose. Pinch the child's nose and then breathe into the child's mouth.

Algorithm

First Aid for a Responsive Infant or Child with a Blocked Airway

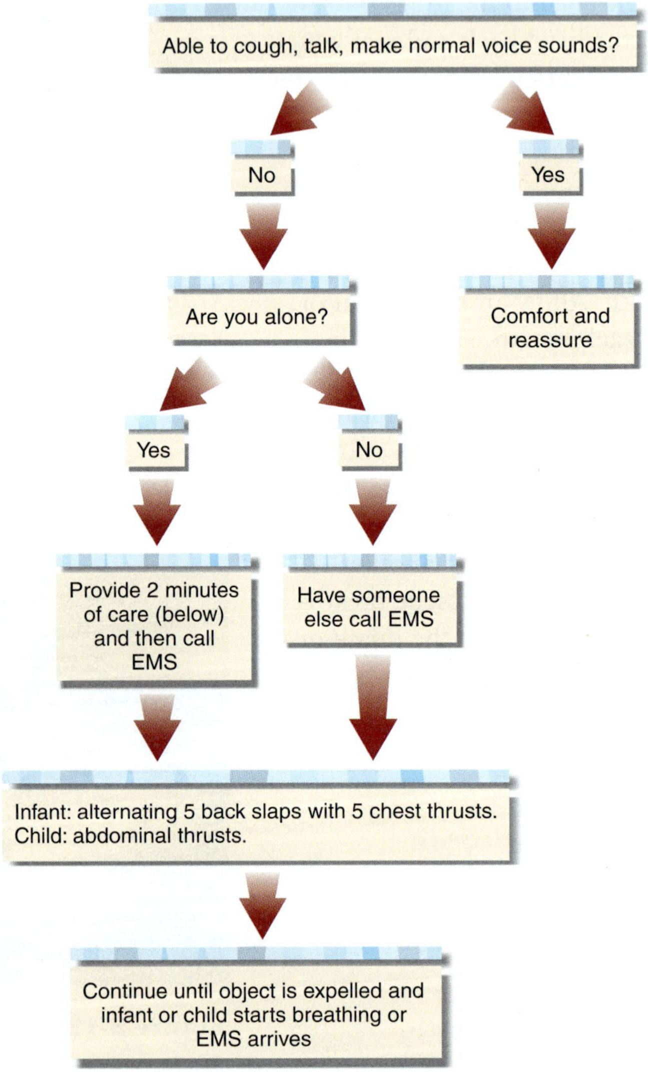

First Aid for an Infant or Child Who is Unconscious/Unresponsive and Not Breathing

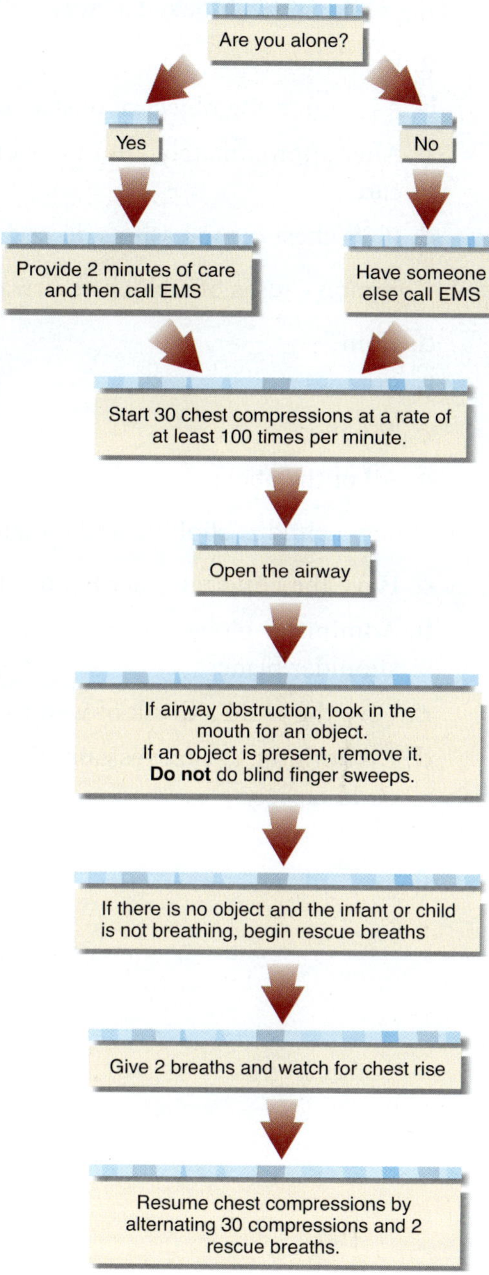

Check Your Knowledge

1. When you are alone and caring for an unresponsive choking child with a blocked airway, call EMS:
   a. Immediately.
   b. As soon as the object of obstruction is removed.
   c. After approximately 2 minutes of performing first aid care.
   d. If 30 chest compressions do not remove the obstruction.
2. Common causes of a blocked airway in children include:
   a. Coin.
   b. Button.
   c. Toy.
   d. All of the above.
3. When a child is choking and coughing hard, you should:
   a. Have the child raise her hands above her head.
   b. Administer blows (slaps) by hand between the child's shoulder blades.
   c. Give the child a drink of water.
   d. Do nothing, except reassure the child and observe the child closely.

Terms

Cardiac arrest	When the heart stops beating.
Nasal flaring	Enlarging of the opening of the nostrils.
Rescue breathing	The act of breathing for a person who is not breathing.
Respiratory arrest	When breathing stops.
Sniffing position	A position children may assume when working hard to breathe; their heads are slightly elevated and they lean forward as if they are sniffing a flower.
Tripod position	The way a child will sit up, placing his arms in front of his chest and out to his side to make the best use of his respiratory muscles.
Universal distress signal	The hands around the throat is the universal distress signal for choking.
Wheezing	A whistling sound made by a child with swelling or blockage of chest tubes.

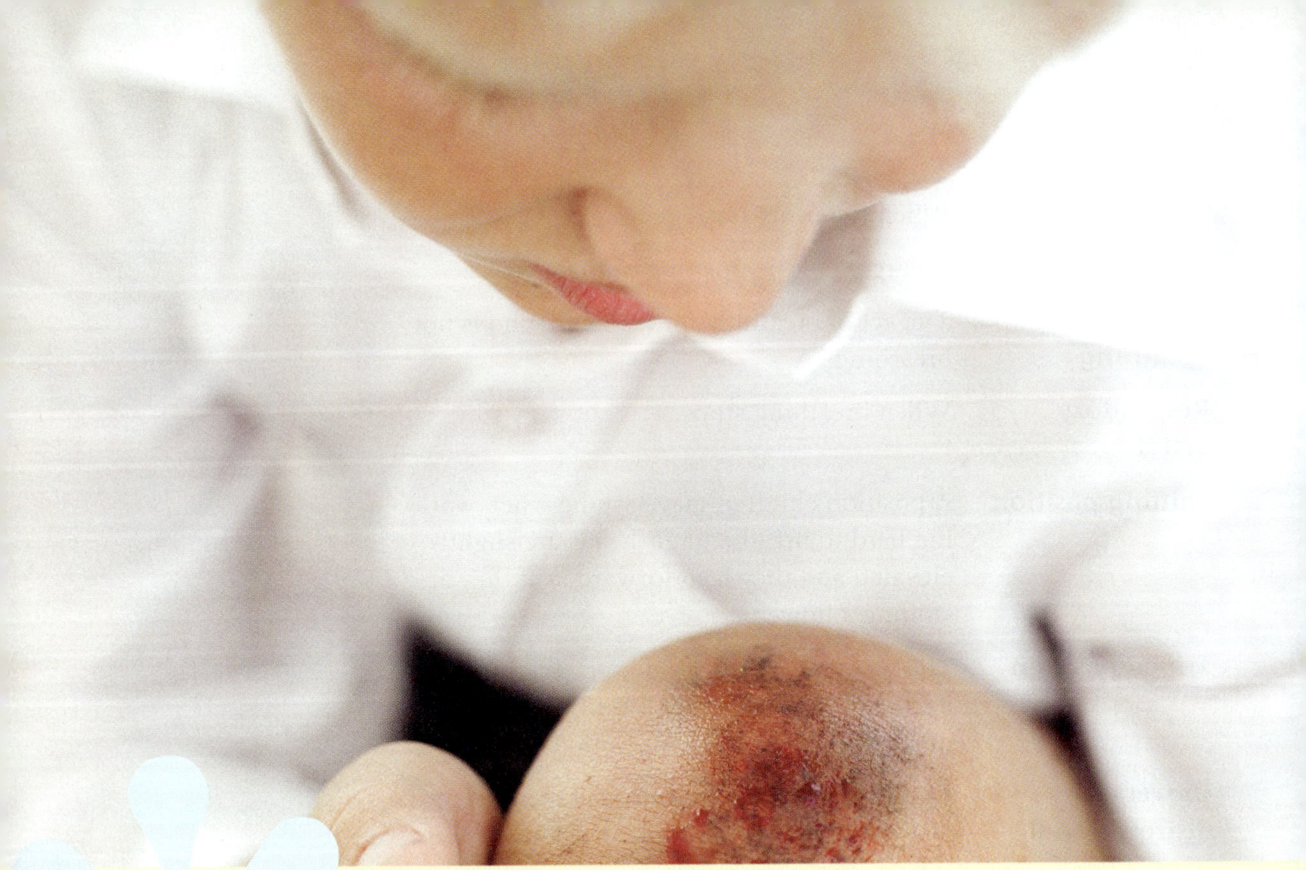

Learning Objectives

The participant will be able to:

- Describe Standard Precautions and Universal Precautions.
- Recognize abrasions, lacerations, and puncture wounds.
- Demonstrate how to apply direct pressure to a bleeding wound.
- Describe the appropriate first aid for abrasions, lacerations, blisters, bruises, and puncture wounds.
- Demonstrate how to control a nosebleed.

Topic 4 Controlling Infection, Bleeding, and Swelling

Controlling Infection

Introduction

Infections are caused by viruses, bacteria, and other germs. Infections can be passed from one person to another. Knowing how germs are transmitted and how to protect against infection while performing first aid will enable you to act wisely and with confidence. While caring for wounds, you need to know how to prevent infection of the wound and how to handle body fluids to protect yourself from infection.

What You Should Know

Controlling the spread of infection requires protecting yourself against exposure to germs and reducing the number of germs in the environment. When the skin has been opened by an injury, germs can enter this opening and start to grow. Reducing the number of germs in a wound helps prevent infection. You can reduce the number of germs by rinsing wounds with soap and running water as soon as possible. You must be sure to control bleeding first, and then rinse out a wound to remove dirt and germs. Generally, except for nosebleeds and wounds that are bleeding freely, prompt rinsing of an open wound with soap and running water is appropriate first aid to reduce the number of germs that can cause infection. The sooner the germs are rinsed out of a wound, the better. Germs multiply very rapidly in a wound and can soon overwhelm the body's defenses against infection.

When body fluids contact an object that others might touch, the body fluids must be removed by cleaning with detergent and rinsing with water. This helps to remove the source of infection, although some germs will remain. To further reduce the number of germs left behind on the visibly clean surface, use a sanitizer. This two-step process makes infection from body fluids unlikely.

Standard Precautions and **Universal Precautions** describe actions developed by the Centers for Disease Control and Prevention (CDC) and the Occupational Safety and Health Administration (OSHA) to help protect people from infections transferred through body fluids. Standard Precautions are the measures required to protect against contact with any type of body fluid, except sweat. Universal Precautions are the protective measures that apply only to blood, and body fluids that might contain blood.

Hand washing after cleaning and sanitizing is essential (**Figure 4-1**). Wearing gloves or using other barriers are not a substitute for washing your hands with soap and running water after a possible exposure to a body fluid. Individuals should wash their hands carefully after possible contact with germs, whether or not barriers were used. Using a barrier reduces, but does not totally eliminate, contact with body fluids.

As mentioned, universal precautions are guidelines designed to protect persons from exposure to potentially infectious diseases spread by blood and body fluids. It is important to protect yourself when handling any body fluid and to treat all fluids as potentially harmful. Remember that universal precautions are designed to protect both the caregiver and the child.

Typically, the minimally accepted universal precautions include wearing protective gloves when treating any ill or injured child. Gloves are meant to provide a barrier between your skin and any potentially harmful body fluid(s).

Additional precautions also include eye protection (goggles) for splashing fluids or face shields (masks) when coughing and sneezing are present.

The need for such precautions has come about with the increased awareness of HIV/AIDS. Human Immunodeficiency Virus (HIV) is a virus that causes Acquired Immune Deficiency Syndrome (AIDS). Children with HIV are considered to be HIV positive and are never "cured" but do not always develop AIDS. Children who are HIV positive can lead normal lives and may never develop AIDS or complications.

HIV is transmitted through body fluids and primarily through sexual intercourse, breastfeeding, childbirth, sharing of needles,

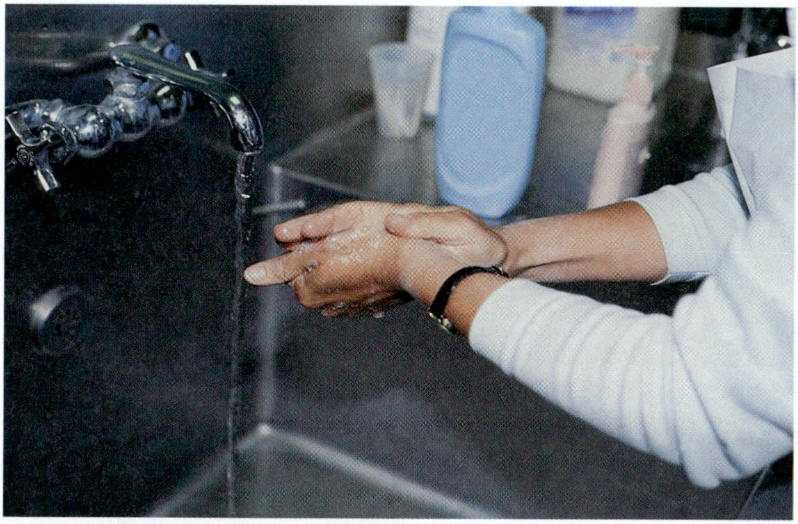

Figure 4-1

Hand washing is essential.

and blood transfusions. HIV is not transmitted by: saliva, tears, sweat, feces or urine; hugging; kissing; shaking hands; insect bites; or sharing toilets with an HIV positive child.

Remember to protect yourself prior to caring for any ill or injured child. Use the universal precautions and you will significantly decrease the risk of exposure to diseases.

First Aid Tip

Reducing contact with germs can help to control the spread of germs and prevent infection. Using the following barriers can help to reduce the exposure of staff and children to germs:

- Non-porous gloves (such as non-latex medical exam gloves or vinyl gloves) (**Figure 4-2**)
- Disposable diaper table paper (required for sanitary diaper changing)
- Disposable towels for cleaning-up and sanitizing surfaces
- Non-porous surfaces that can be cleaned and sanitized
- Clothing to prevent contact of your skin with the body fluids of someone else, especially when blood might be involved and you do not have gloves
- Plastic bags to store contaminated articles until they can be thrown away or sanitized

Figure 4-2

Gloves are a barrier against germs.

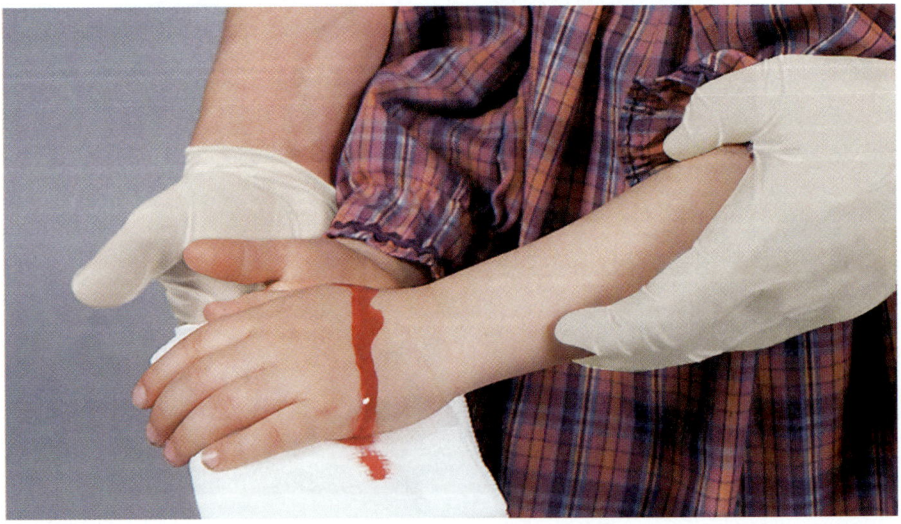

What You Should Look For

When a child has been injured, you need to look for places where the skin has been cut or where tissues have been injured. Tissue injury comes from some force pressing hard on a body part, twisting or pinching the skin or other tissues. Bleeding, bruising, swelling, or pain may indicate tissue injury. If the injury has opened the skin, you may come in contact with blood.

Having cuts or open sores on your own hands increases your risk of getting an infection from contact with germs from surfaces and from a child's body fluids. If you have cuts or sores on your hands, you need to protect these openings with clean coverings (e.g., a bandage) and wear non-porous gloves when handling body fluids.

Did You Know?

For most persons likely to be exposed to blood, Universal Precautions require that they are provided the opportunity to be protected by vaccination against infection by the hepatitis B virus. National health experts recommend vaccination for hepatitis B for all children and for those adults who might give first aid.

What You Should Do

Procedure for Standard Precautions When Cleaning Up Body Fluids

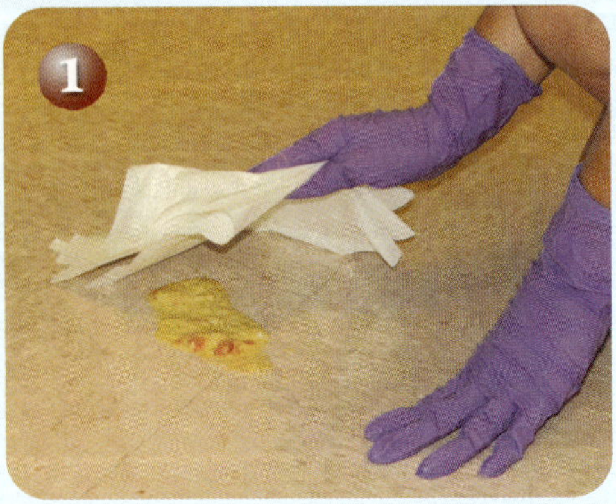

1 Use non-porous gloves and whatever tools (e.g., paper towels, tissues, rags, mop) you have to wipe up the spill. Try to use disposable tools to minimize the need to do further cleaning and sanitizing. Avoid spreading the spilled body fluid.

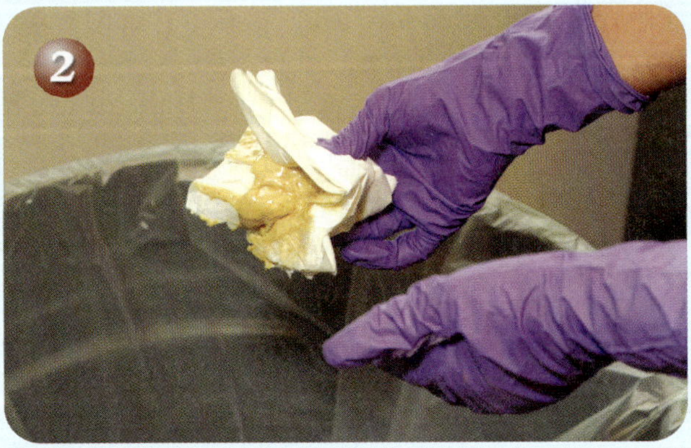

2 Put all tools (e.g., paper towels, tissues, rags, mops) that you used to wipe up the spill into a plastic-lined receptacle for disposal or to clean and sanitize later.

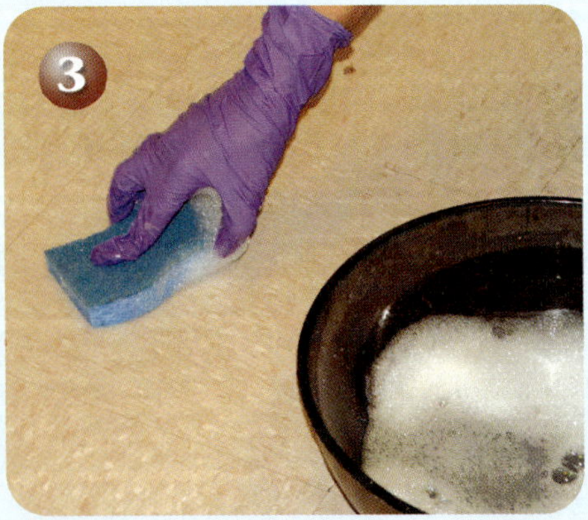

3 Use a detergent to clean all surfaces in contact with the spill, including floors and rugs.

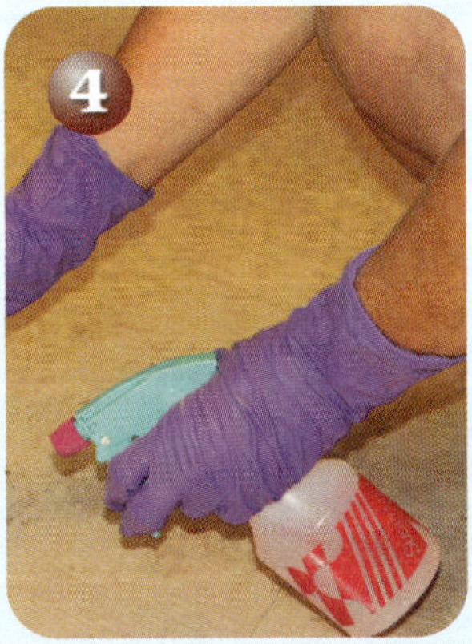

4 Rinse cleaned surfaces with water.

Procedure for Standard Precautions When Cleaning Up Body Fluids (cont.)

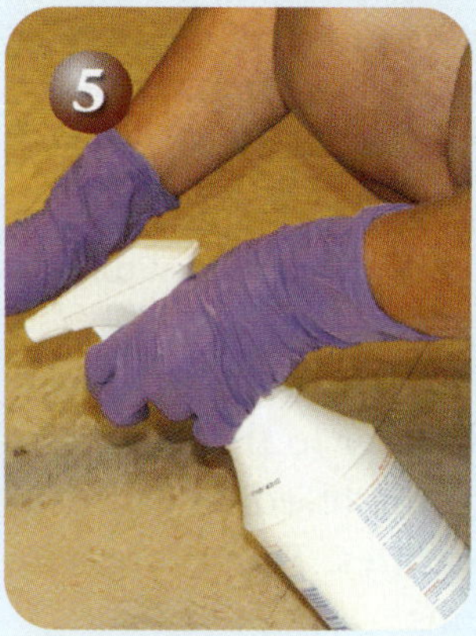

5 Apply a sanitizing solution, following the manufacturer's instructions on the label. (An inexpensive and effective sanitizing solution can be made by diluting 1/4 cup of household bleach mixed with 1 gallon of water, or 1 tablespoon of bleach to 1 quart of water. This solution must be left in contact with the surface for at least 2 minutes.)

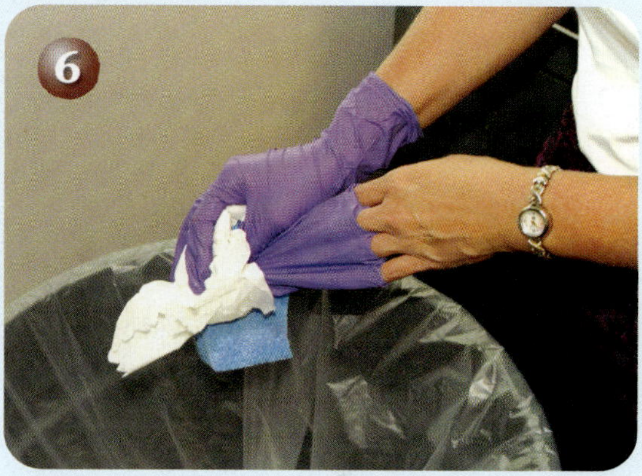

6 Put contaminated cleaning material in a plastic bag with a secure tie for disposal. This can be the same plastic bag you used for the tools from wiping up the spill.

Bleeding

What You Should Know

When the skin is cut and a blood vessel of any size is broken, bleeding occurs. The seriousness of the injury is determined by the depth of the cut, the type of blood vessels damaged, and the amount of bleeding that occurs. The most severe bleeding is from **arteries**, which are large, deep, and well-protected blood vessels. Injury to an artery is serious. Large amounts of blood can be lost from arteries in a short amount of time. If arterial bleeding is not controlled, it can be life-threatening. Apply pressure by pushing with your hand over the injured area to stop the flow of blood. Applying pressure to a wound with your hand or with a firmly applied dressing is called **direct pressure**.

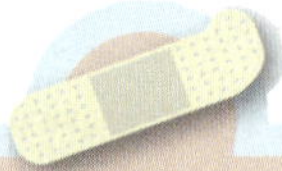

First Aid Tip

Most bleeding that occurs in children is not life-threatening. Usually, bleeding from small blood vessels stops quickly. Do not panic when you see what seems to be a lot of blood coming from a cut anywhere on the head or face. Since blood is a vivid red color, a little blood may look like a larger volume than it really is. Bleeding that does not stop by itself within a minute or so requires first aid care to stop the bleeding before larger amounts of blood are lost.

Veins are blood vessels that are located closer to the surface of the skin. Although a vein can bleed heavily, the bleeding can usually be controlled with simple first aid measures. Direct pressure works well for controlling bleeding from veins.

Tiny blood vessels located throughout the body are called **capillaries.** There are hundreds of thousands of capillaries throughout the body. When capillaries are broken, bleeding is easy to control. Direct pressure stops bleeding from capillaries quickly.

Some parts of the body have more blood vessels than others. For example, the head and face have more blood vessels in a given area than the finger. That is why a cut on the head or face bleeds more than a cut on a finger.

Injuries that occur deep in the chest, abdomen, or in the brain may be associated with bleeding in tissues far below the skin. This type of injury is called **internal bleeding.** The symptoms of internal bleeding vary with the type of injury and the body part involved. Usually, the person with internal bleeding feels severe pain and looks very ill. If you suspect that a child may have internal bleeding, call EMS immediately. Attempt to keep the child calm while waiting for EMS to arrive.

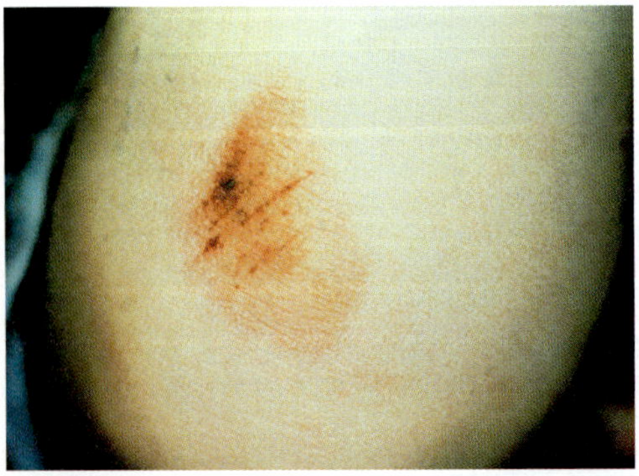

Figure 4-3

Abrasion.

If the skin is broken, the wound is called an **open wound.** Common types of open wounds include scrapes (abrasions), cuts (lacerations), broken blisters, punctures, and nosebleeds.

Abrasions occur when the top layer of skin is removed, with little blood loss (**Figure 4-3**). Even though abrasions are not life-threatening, infection can occur. Abrasions can be quite painful. Many nerve endings may be exposed with the loss of the top layer of skin. An example of an abrasion is a scraped knee.

A **laceration** is a cut, which can be jagged or smooth (**Figure 4-4**). Lacerations may be superficial or deep, large or small. An example of a laceration is a cut from a knife, broken glass, or a paper cut.

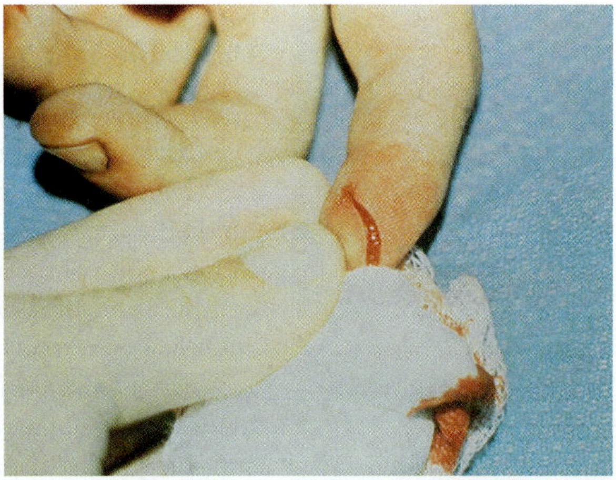

Figure 4-4

Laceration.

A **blister** is a collection of fluid in a bubble underneath the skin. These can be small or large. Generally, if the skin over a blister is not broken, the fluid inside the blister is sterile.

A **puncture** is a small hole made in the skin, which may be either deep or shallow. Puncture wounds usually bleed very little. Puncture wounds have a high risk of infection because it is hard to wash out the germs in the hole that the penetrating object made in the skin. An example of a puncture wound is a splinter.

An avulsion is a piece of skin torn loose and hanging from the body. An amputation is the cutting or tearing off of a body part. Avulsions and amputations, while rare, can occur and should be handled like most other bleeding wounds. Be sure to use universal precautions to minimize the risk of infection. Call EMS and control the bleeding and remember to care for the both the exposed part and the avulsed or amputated part.

A nosebleed is bleeding from the nose. Nosebleeds occur more frequently in winter when allergies, respiratory infections, or dry air are associated with itching and picking of the nose. Blowing the nose too hard or hitting the nose can also cause nosebleeds.

If a blood vessel breaks in the nostril, then blood runs out of the nostril. Tilting the child's head back or lying the child down may make the blood stop running out of the nostril, but it does not stop the bleeding. Some people mistakenly think they can stop a nosebleed by tipping the head back. You see less blood when the child lies down or tilts his head back because the blood drips down the

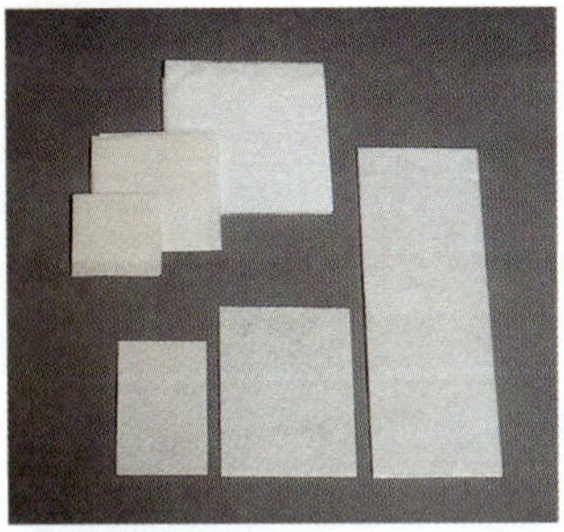

Figure 4-5

Dressing.

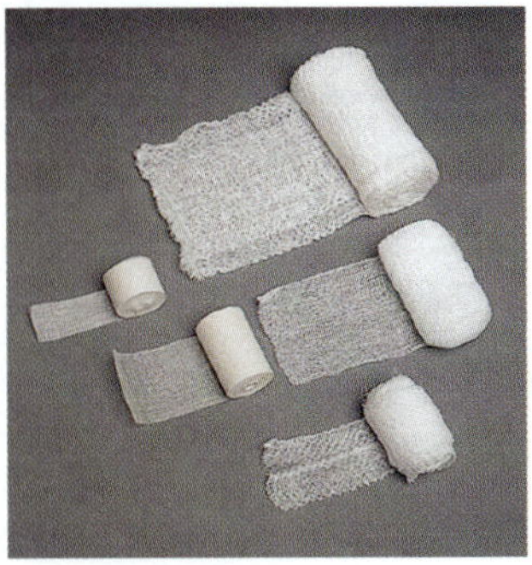

Figure 4-6

Bandage.

back of the child's throat and the child swallows it. Swallowed blood upsets the stomach and may lead to vomiting. The stress of vomiting may make the nosebleed worse.

Open wounds may require dressings and bandages. A **dressing** is a clean covering placed over a wound (**Figure 4-5**). A **bandage** holds the dressing in place and also can be used to apply pressure to help control bleeding (**Figure 4-6**). An **adhesive bandage** is a combination of a dressing and a bandage. Commercial dressings, such as gauze pads, nonstick gauze pads, and adhesive bandages come in a variety of sizes. Sterile, commercially prepared, individually wrapped gauze pads are lint-free and easy to store in first aid supplies. Rolls of gauze can be used on any part of the body and come in various widths.

What You Should Look For

- Look carefully and see where the blood is coming from or where it seems to be accumulating under the skin. Children who have only a small cut under the top lip may have blood on their lips and tongue as well as on their shirts. Until you find the source of the blood, you might think that the lip, tongue, or face has been cut.
- Check if the blood is still flowing or if the flow has stopped.
- Observe whether the child who has had a big fall seems to be in pain or looks very ill. This may be a sign of internal bleeding.

Did You Know

Dressings that have a plastic back keep blood from leaking through to the outside. However, small plastic-backed dressings can be serious choking hazards for children under 3 years of age. A young child may remove the plastic-backed dressing from a wound and put the dressing in his mouth. If the plastic dressing gets positioned across an airway, the child may not be able to breathe. Avoid plastic-backed dressings for children under 3 years of age. Use fabric bandages and dressings instead.

What You Should Do

The Eight Steps in Pediatric First Aid:

1 Survey the Scene

Take a brief moment to perform a scene survey to ensure that the scene is safe, to find out who is involved, and to determine what happened.

2 Hands-off ABCs

As you approach the child, perform the hands-off ABCs (Appearance, Breathing, and Circulation) to determine if EMS should be called. It should take 15 to 30 seconds or less.

3 Supervise

Immediately ensure that any other children near the scene are properly supervised.

4 Hands-on ABCDEs

Perform the hands-on ABCDEs (Appearance, Breathing, Circulation, Disability, and Everything else) to determine if EMS should be called and what first aid care is needed.

5 First Aid Care

Provide first aid care appropriate to the injury or illness.

6 Notify

As soon as possible, notify the child's parent(s) or legal guardian(s).

7 Debrief

As soon as possible, talk with the child who received first aid about any concerns he or she may have, and talk with other children who witnessed the injury and first aid procedures.

8 Document

Complete an incident report form.

What You Should Do

First Aid Care for an Open Wound (scrapes, cuts, tears, avulsions, amputations of body tissues)

1. Follow Standard Precautions. Use a barrier between your skin and the bleeding wound. Protect your hand with a glove, a wad of toweling paper, or any other clean material that is available while you apply pressure to the wound.

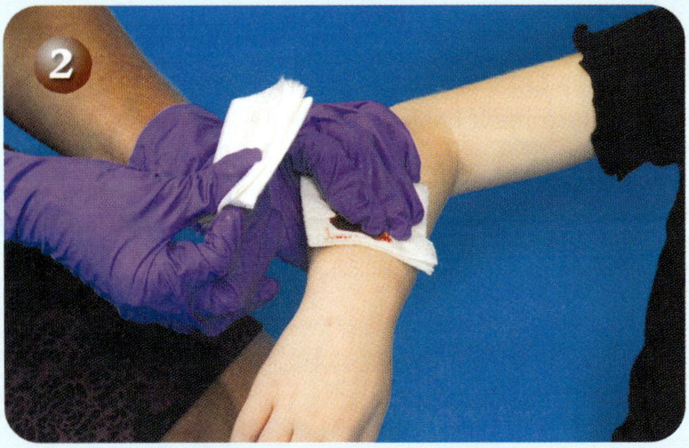

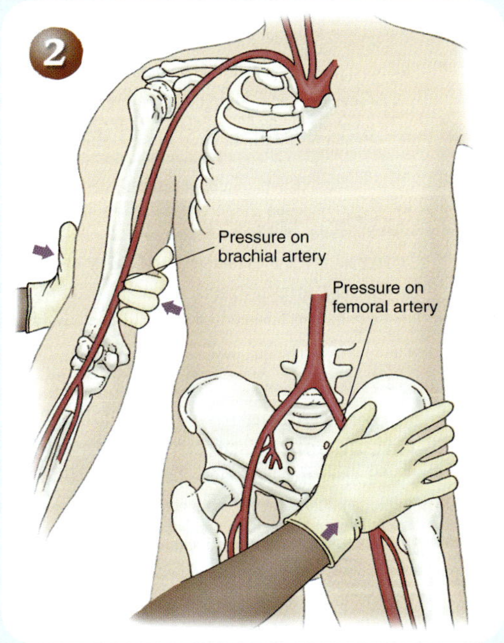

2. Apply direct pressure with your fingers or the palm of your hand to the spot that is bleeding until the bleeding stops. Usually, bleeding will stop after 1 to 2 minutes of direct pressure. If you can control bleeding easily, wash the wound with soap and clean, running water, apply a bandage and follow up with the parent(s) or legal guardian(s). If bleeding is difficult to control, keep pressure on the wound for at least 5 minutes. If blood is seeping through the dressings while you apply pressure, do not remove the dressing that is in direct contact with the wound. Removing the dressing from contact with the wound may remove a clot that is forming to plug up the blood vessel that is bleeding. Apply additional dressings as needed. If the bleeding continues, apply pressure to one of the four pressure points. Pressure points are located in each of the upper arms and groin area of each leg. Applying pressure to these areas will slow the blood flow to the wound.

First Aid Care for an Open Wound (cont.)

2a Avulsed parts should be allowed to remain intact and should be placed back in its normal position, unless dirt and debris are in the wound. Care for avulsed parts in the same manner as other open wounds. Amputated parts should be kept dry and placed on ice. The part should not be submerged in ice or water, but should be wrapped in a clean, dry, sterile dressing and be put in a plastic bag and placed on ice.

3 If the bleeding continues or starts again after 5 minutes of sustained direct pressure, call EMS.

4 Wipe up the spill and sanitize the surfaces following Standard Precautions.

5 If the wound is very dirty and the child has not had a tetanus booster in the past 5 years, the child may need to see a medical professional, as a booster may be needed.

First Aid Tip

- A wound should be evaluated by a medical professional if it will not stay closed by itself, or requires 5 minutes of sustained direct pressure to control bleeding. The wound may require stitches.
- The edges of cuts longer than ½ inch may gap. These need to be managed by a medical professional who will use stitches, tape, or some other special way to keep the edges of the skin together while the wound heals. To prevent infection and get the best healing, stitches are applied as soon as possible—generally within 6 hours of the injury.
- Prompt and proper cleaning, followed by closing of an open wound, reduces the risk of infection, promotes healing, and decreases scarring.
- A child can suck on a popsicle to apply cold and pressure to cuts on lips or under the tongue, or to injured teeth.

What You Should Do

First Aid Care for Blisters

1. Protect blisters with a bandage. The bandage will help keep the blister from opening for as long as possible while the injured tissues under the blister heal.

2. Recommend to the parent(s) or legal guardian(s) that they should arrange for blisters that are larger than a quarter to be evaluated by a medical professional.

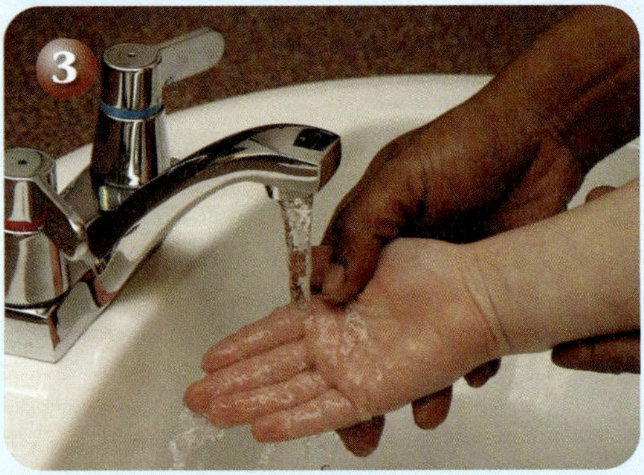

3. If the blister opens, clean it with water and care for it in the same way you treat an open wound.

What You Should Do

First Aid Care for Punctures, Including Splinters

1. With parental consent, pull out small objects you can grasp easily, (e.g., a wood splinter or staple) with clean tweezers. If you cannot get a small object out easily, or if the object is large, or is deeply embedded, medical help is needed. Call EMS if the penetrating object is large (e.g., a knife, stick, or an object embedded deeply below the skin). Do not pull out or move such an object. If appropriate, apply a bandage to keep the object from moving around or doing further damage.

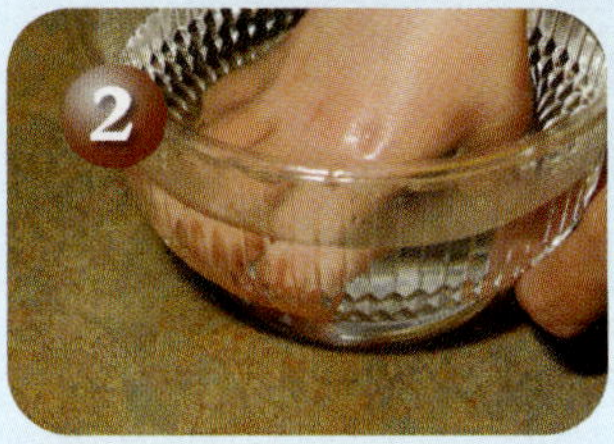

2. Soak the wound in clean water.

3. For wounds where the object has been removed, soak the wound again in clean water and then bandage the wound loosely or leave it without a bandage.

4. If the object was very dirty and it has been more than 5 years since the child's last tetanus booster, the child may need to see a medical professional as a booster may be needed.

What You Should Do

First Aid Care for Nosebleeds

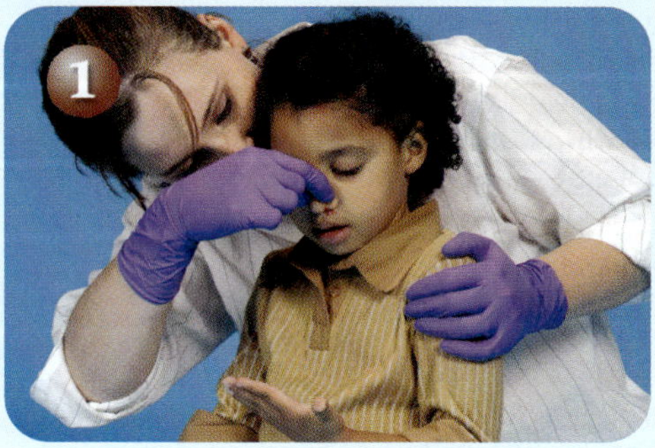

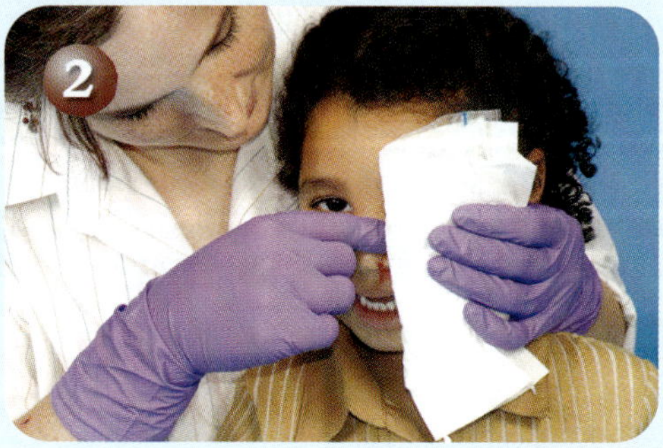

1. Keep the child sitting up.

2. Follow Standard Precautions. Use the thumb and a finger of one hand to pinch all of the soft parts of the nose together.

3. Gently press the pinched nose against the bones of the face.

4. Hold that position for a full 5 minutes. Do not peek to see if bleeding has stopped.

5. If you can, apply ice to the child's nose and cheeks using a plastic bag of ice or frozen vegetables wrapped in a cloth while you apply the pressure to the nose.

6. After 5 minutes of pressure, gently release the nose to avoid restarting the nosebleed. A sudden rush of blood re-entering the damaged blood vessel in the nose could dislodge the clot that formed while you kept the nose pinched and pressed against the face. If bleeding starts again, reapply the pressure, but for longer this time.

7. Have the child do a quiet activity for at least 30 minutes after the nosebleed stops, to avoid restarting the bleeding.

8. Avoid blowing the child's nose after stopping the nosebleed. Blowing the nose could dislodge the clot. If the child can do so easily, have the child blow out the excess blood right before you apply pressure so there will be less blood in the nose after the bleeding has been stopped. Since the blood forms scabs that can be itchy, large amounts of blood left in the nose may lead the child to pick and start the bleeding again.

9. Call EMS or get medical help if a nosebleed cannot be controlled.

Did You Know

Tetanus is a disease that is sometimes called "lockjaw." Bacteria that can cause tetanus live in the soil, dust, and in human and animal feces. These bacteria enter the body through a dirty wound and the resulting tetanus causes strong spasms in the back, legs, arms, and jaw (lockjaw). The disease is usually fatal, but routine and periodic tetanus vaccinations have made most people in the US immune to tetanus. Vaccination teaches the immune system of the body to develop protection against future exposure to tetanus. Children should receive routine tetanus shots at 2 months, 4 months, 6 months, 12 to 15 months, 4 to 6 years of age and every 10 years thereafter throughout life. An extra dose is given at the time of injury only if a wound is particularly dirty and it has been at least 5 years since the last booster.

Swelling

What You Should Know

With a **closed wound** the skin is not broken, but the tissue and blood vessels underneath the skin's surface are crushed, causing bleeding within a confined area. Closed wounds include bruises. Active children, especially those who engage in vigorous play, will often have bruises (**Figure 4-7**). Swelling can also occur with a closed wound.

Initially, a bruised area is red and swollen and then gradually turns blue or purple. As the blood is absorbed over the next few days, the area turns yellow and fades as it heals.

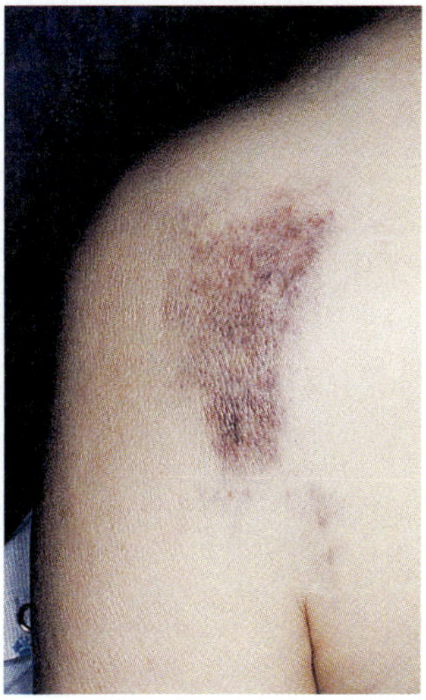

Figure 4-7

Bruise.

Did You Know

The air tends to be very dry in the winter months in cold climates, in air conditioned environments, and in some desert climates. Adding moisture to dry air with a humidifier or vaporizer helps to reduce the risk of nosebleeds. When nosebleeds are a problem, some health care professionals encourage families to put saline nasal mist spray or some petroleum jelly in the child's nasal openings to help protect the delicate nasal tissues from harsh, dry air. This can only be done with the permission of the parent(s) or legal guardian(s).

First Aid Tip

When a body part has been crushed, the damage may be more severe than is immediately apparent. Swelling from a crush injury can collapse the walls of blood vessels, pinching them and cutting off the necessary blood supply to tissues. If this condition continues, the tissues die. A medical professional must always evaluate crush injuries, even if they do not look severe.

What You Should Look For

- Check to see what caused the injury.
- Compare the injured part of the body with the same body part of the opposite side to see if there is swelling.
- Touch the skin to see if the skin feels tense.
- Look for discoloration of the skin over the injured area.
- If a body part was caught between two hard surfaces and squeezed or twisted, there may be a crush injury. If you have any suspicion that a crush injury occurred, proceed as if this is a potentially serious problem and arrange for the child to be evaluated by a medical professional.

What You Should Do

First Aid Care for Bruises and Swelling

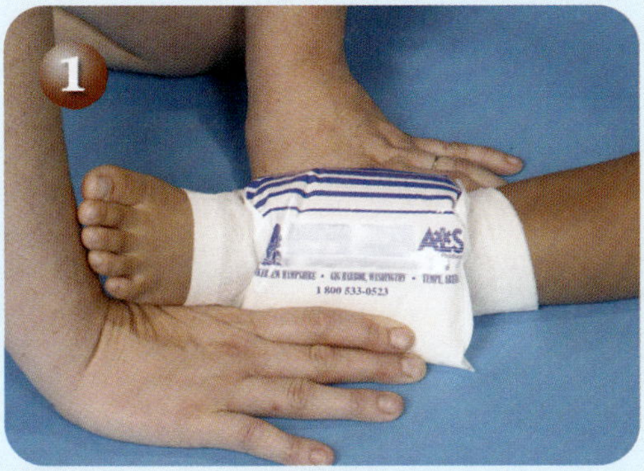

1. To control swelling, apply cold using ice, a bag of frozen vegetables, or a cold pack that is wrapped in a towel. Do not apply a frozen object directly against the skin because extreme cold may cause further injury.

2. Call EMS or get medical help if there is continued pain or swelling, or the child has had a crush injury.

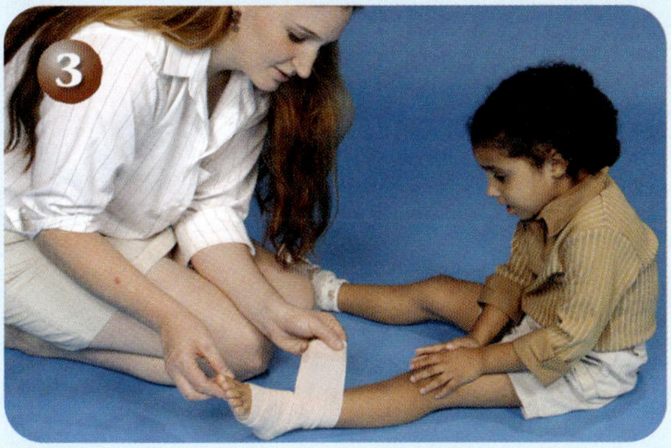

3. Stretchy rolled gauze or elastic bandages can be applied to put pressure on a bruised or a swollen area. They can also help to hold cold packs in place. If you use these bandages, leave the tips of fingers and toes exposed so that you can tell if the body part is wrapped too tightly. Check for changes in color, temperature, and whether the fingers or toes lose their pink color. The fingers or toes should have normal skin color and feel warm to the touch.

4. Elevate the injury unless you suspect a broken bone or a spinal injury. Moving a child with a broken bone or a spinal injury can cause more injury to occur (see Musculoskeletal Injuries).

Algorithm

First Aid for Bleeding

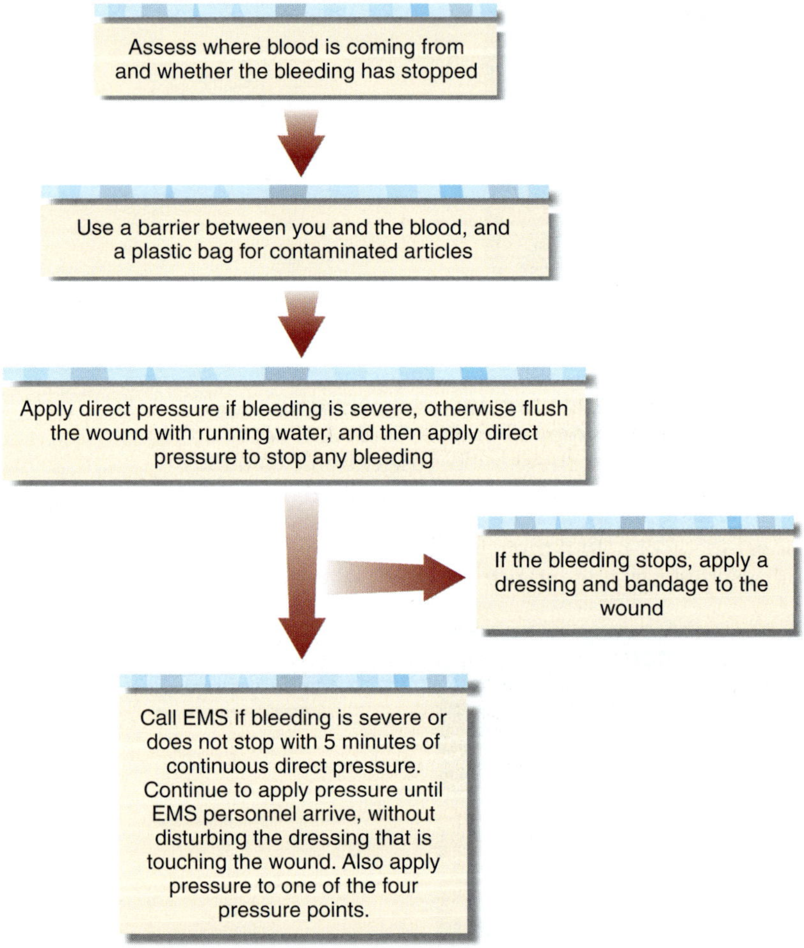

Check Your Knowledge

1. To reduce the risk of infection, clean small wounds by:

- **a.** Rubbing the dirt out with a soapy wash cloth.
- **b.** Pouring alcohol on the injured area.
- **c.** Flushing the injured area with running water.
- **d.** Wiping the wound with a commercially packaged antiseptic wipe.

2. To control severe bleeding:

- **a.** Place firm, direct pressure on the wound.
- **b.** Put ice directly on the wound.
- **c.** Apply a tourniquet.
- **d.** Hold the injured part up.

3. To control swelling in an injured part:

- **a.** Put ice directly on the injury.
- **b.** Place warm compresses on the injured body part.
- **c.** Apply cold, wrap, and elevate the injured body part.
- **d.** Place the injured part in a splint.

4. To control a nosebleed:

- **a.** Have the child tilt his head back.
- **b.** Have the child lie down.
- **c.** Ask the child to blow his nose until the bleeding stops.
- **d.** Pinch the soft parts of the nose and press against the bones of the face.

Terms

Abrasions	Open wounds that occur when the top layer of skin is removed, with little blood loss.
Adhesive bandage	Combination of a dressing and a bandage.
Arteries	Large, deep, and well-protected blood vessels. Arteries carry blood away from the heart to all parts of the body.
Bandage	Holds the dressing in place and also can be used to apply pressure to help control bleeding.
Blister	A collection of fluid in a bubble underneath the skin.
Capillaries	Tiny blood vessels located throughout the body.
Closed wound	Type of wound where the skin is not broken, but the tissue and blood vessels underneath the skin's surface are crushed, causing bleeding within a confined area.
Direct pressure	Applying pressure to a wound with your hand or with a firmly applied dressing.

Dressing	A clean covering placed over a wound.
Internal bleeding	Injuries that occur deep in the chest, abdomen, or in the brain may be associated with bleeding in tissues far below the skin.
Laceration	A cut, which could be jagged or smooth.
Open wound	An injury that breaks the skin.
Puncture	A small hole made in the skin, which may be either deep or shallow.
Standard Precautions	Measures required to protect against contact with any body fluids that might contain blood. Precautions include cleaning and sanitizing surfaces that have come in contact with any type of body fluids (except sweat) and hand washing.
Universal Precautions	Protective measures that apply to blood, bodily fluids that might contain blood, and sexual secretions. They do not apply to feces, nasal secretions, sputum, sweat, tears, urine, and vomitus.
Veins	Blood vessels that carry blood back to the heart.

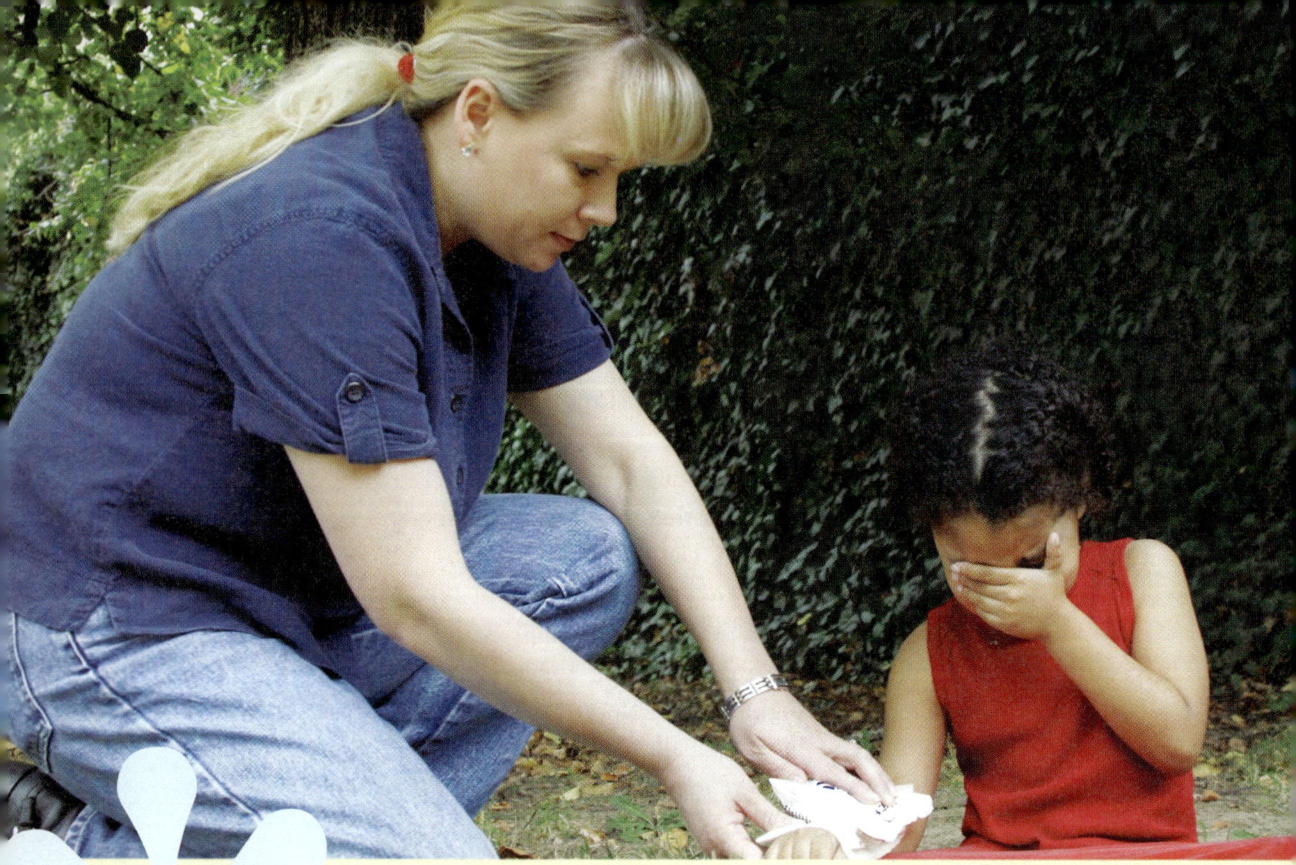

Learning Objectives

The participant will be able to:

- Define closed and open fracture.
- Describe how to use DOTS (Deformity, Open injury, Tenderness, and Swelling) to assess a musculoskeletal injury.
- Describe how to use RICE (Rest, Ice, Compression, Elevation) to treat a minor musculoskeletal injury.
- Identify the appropriate response to suspected:
  a. Broken bones (fractures)
  b. Dislocations
  c. Sprains
  d. Injuries to the spine

Topic

5

Bone, Joint, and Muscle Injuries

Bone, Joint, and Muscle Injuries

Introduction

The bones and joints of young children are generally more flexible than those of adults. Unlike adults, children rarely strain or tear muscles and ligaments while stretching, bending, or running. However, young children are more prone to dislocation of the joints than adults, especially dislocation of the elbow. Due to their impulsive behavior, children frequently experience broken bones and bruises. Spinal injuries involve the bones and joints of the spine, muscles that surround the spine, or the spinal cord and nerves. Collectively, bones, joints, and muscles are called the **musculoskeletal system.**

What You Should Know

A **fracture** is a broken bone. Any bone in the body can be fractured, including those of the limbs, trunk, and spine. A fracture can be a partial break or a complete break in the bone. The surrounding muscles, nerves, and blood vessels can also be damaged when the bone is fractured.

Fractures are common in children. Fortunately, children's bones heal more rapidly after a fracture than those of adults. Although healing is usually complete, sometimes a fracture can cause trouble with growth or full range of motion in the part of the body where the bone was broken.

A **closed fracture** occurs when the skin is not broken at the location of the fracture. An **open fracture** occurs when there is an open wound over the fracture. The wound can occur either from the broken edge of the bone cutting through the tissues and skin, or from the force that broke the bone (**Figure 5-1**). The event of blood loss is equal in open and closed fractures, but the blood loss is more obvious in open fractures and there is a greater chance of infection.

A **dislocation** is the separation of a bone from a joint. In children, dislocations commonly happen to fingers and elbows, and are

Figure 5-1

Closed fracture (A), open fracture (B).

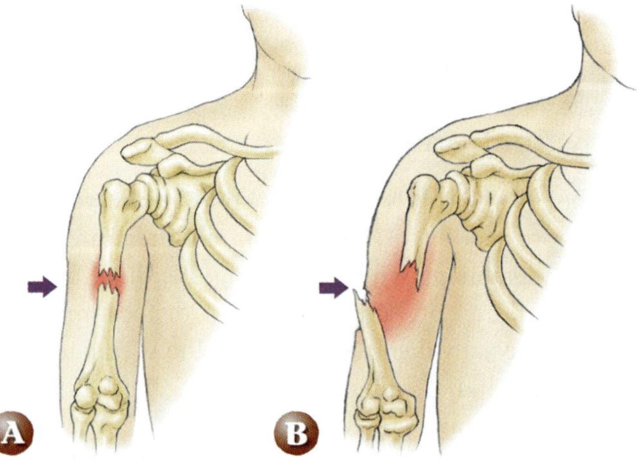

not always obvious. It takes only a small amount of force to dislocate a child's bone. A quick tug on a child's hand to prevent the child from stepping into the street or to protect against a stumble can be enough to dislocate an elbow. Infants and young children should not be picked up by their hands or wrists (**Figure 5-2**).

Sometimes a dislocated bone will go back into the socket by itself right away, but often a medical professional will need to return the bone to its proper position. Loss of movement of the joint causes pain if the bone remains dislocated.

A **sprain** is an injury that occurs when the tissues that hold the joints together (**ligaments**) are stretched beyond their limits. A **strain** occurs when a force stretches a muscle or muscles beyond their limits. Sprains are uncommon in young children but begin to occur in children as they progress through grade school, and their joints become more like adult joints.

At the time of the injury, most children do not want to move a body part that has a fractured bone or a significantly hurt muscle or joint. The injury causes pain and muscle spasm and generally makes children hold the injured body part still. Children may "splint" their own injured body part by holding it against their body or by just holding the body part very still.

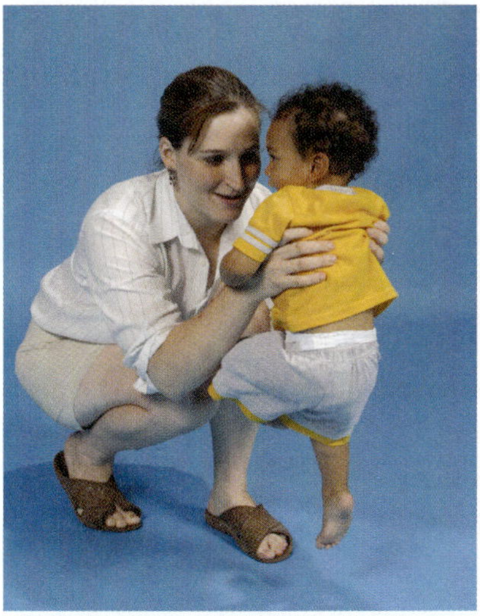

Figure 5-2

Lift children under their arms, not by hands or wrists.

It is not necessary for someone giving first aid to figure out whether there is a fracture, dislocation, sprain, or strain. First aid is the same for any of these injuries. The role of the person giving first aid is to recognize that the child has a potentially serious injury and then use techniques that keep the injured part from moving until a medical professional can evaluate the injury.

What You Should Look For

You should suspect a child may have a musculoskeletal injury based on your initial survey of the scene. If a child has fallen or been struck by some force, some injury to muscles, bones, or joints might have occurred. As you approach the child and are doing your hands-off ABCs, you can observe whether the child is in pain or seems to be holding some body part still in an unnatural way. If a bone, joint, or muscle injury has occurred, the child will complain of pain at the injury site. Even if the child is crying, you can try to get the child to point to where it hurts. Asking the child to point to the spot that hurts helps distract the child from the intensity of the pain and helps you avoid jumping to wrong conclusion about what body part has been hurt. It can be hard to figure out where the injury is located when you see the child crying or refusing to move. The child may be holding an uninjured part to keep the injured part still. Children figure out within seconds that avoiding movement of an injured part reduces the pain.

When dealing with bone, joint, and muscle injuries, use the mnemonic **DOTS (Deformity, Open injury, Tenderness, Swelling)** to assess the extent of the injury.

- Deformity is when a bone is broken and causes an abnormal shape.
- Open injuries or wounds are a break in the skin.
- Tenderness is sensitivity to touch.
- Swelling is the body's response to injury that makes the area look larger than usual.

When muscles, bones, or joints are injured, blood and other fluids collect around the injury. This accumulation of fluid causes swelling. Sometimes a break in the bone results in an unnatural shape or bend of the body part. This unnatural appearance is called a deformity. You can recognize a deformity from your assessment of appearance when you do the hands-off ABCs and hands-on ABCDEs. To detect a deformity, compare the injured body part with the uninjured side. Remember that loss of movement tells you that a bone, muscle, or joint injury may have occurred. The child may be able to move the injured part slightly, but not have full range of motion. In the hands-on ABCDEs, this loss of function is the "D" for disability.

What You Should Do

The Eight Steps in Pediatric First Aid:

1 Survey the Scene

Take a brief moment to perform a scene survey to ensure that the scene is safe, to find out who is involved, and to determine what happened.

2 Hands-off ABCs

As you approach the child, perform the hands-off ABCs (Appearance, Breathing, and Circulation) to determine if EMS should be called. It should take 15 to 30 seconds or less.

3 Supervise

Immediately ensure that any other children near the scene are properly supervised.

4 Hands-on ABCDEs

Perform the hands-on ABCDEs (Appearance, Breathing, Circulation, Disability, and Everything else) to determine if EMS should be called and what first aid care is needed.

5 First Aid Care

Provide first aid care appropriate to the injury or illness.

6 Notify

As soon as possible, notify the child's parent(s) or legal guardian(s).

7 Debrief

As soon as possible, talk with the child who received first aid about any concerns he or she may have, and talk with other children who witnessed the injury and first aid procedures.

8 Document

Complete an incident report form.

What You Should Do

First Aid for Bone, Joint, and Muscle Injuries

First aid and subsequent care for musculoskeletal injuries are known by the mnemonic **RICE (Rest, Ice, Compression, and Elevation)**. If the child can move the body part and it only hurts a little bit, the injury is often minor. Otherwise, a medical professional should evaluate the injury to decide what care is appropriate. Minor injuries can be managed with the measures indicated by RICE.

1. Rest. Have the child assume a comfortable position (e.g., sitting or lying down). Pain is the body's way of indicating that a problem exists. If movement of an injured body part is painful, the child should not be urged to move it.
2. Ice. Cover the injury with a cloth and apply ice or a cold pack for periods of 20 to 30 minutes every 2 to 3 hours for the first 24 to 48 hours. This reduces pain, bleeding, and swelling. Having a cloth between the ice and

the skin protects the skin from extreme cold. An elastic bandage is a good way to hold the ice or cold pack in place. Continuous use of ice or direct contact of ice with the skin can damage the tissue (**Figure 5-3A**).

3. Compression. You can use an elastic bandage to compress the injured area. This limits the collection of blood and other fluids. Start a few inches below and end several inches above the injury. Wrap upward toward the heart in a spiral manner. Use firm, even pressure, making sure you do not wrap too tightly. If the child complains that the fin-

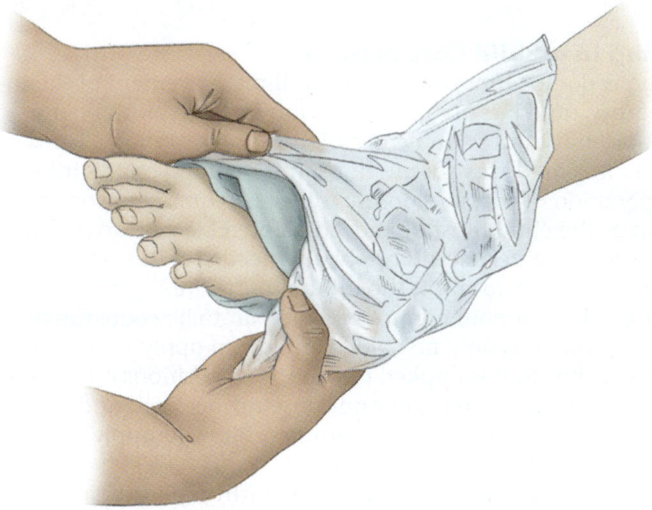

Figure 5-3A

RICE. A. Ice.

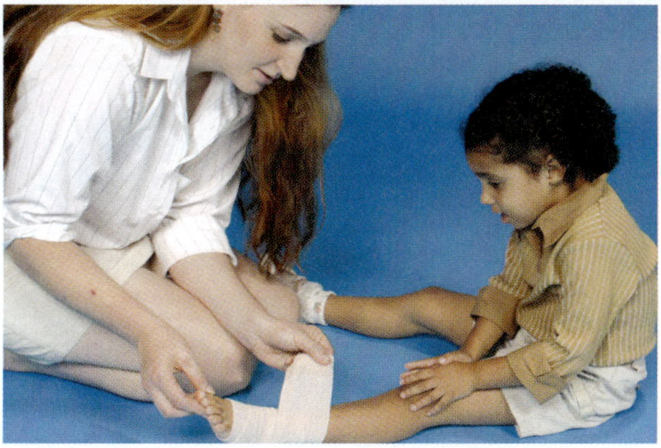

Figure 5-3B

RICE.
B. Compression.

First Aid Tip

- Do not wrap a compression bandage too tightly.
- Assess the color of the area below the bandage to assure that the bandage is not too tight.
- Always protect the skin by wrapping the ice in a thin cloth.
- Do not use ice for longer than 20 to 30 minutes at a time because it can damage the tissue.

gers or toes are cold, tingling, or becoming numb, loosen the bandage. Remove the elastic bandage only when applying ice (**Figure 5-3B**).

4. Elevation. Elevate the injury above the level of the heart by placing the injured limb on several pillows. This limits blood flow to the injury and reduces swelling.

Did You Know

Splinting in a Child Care Setting

Splinting is doing what is necessary to limit movement of the injured part as much as possible. Knowing how to splint a bone, muscle, or joint injury can be useful in many situations. However, teachers and caregivers should not splint a young child's injury unless application of pressure on the injury is required to control bleeding or the child must be moved before EMS can arrive. Instead, EMS personnel should apply any needed splint. The reasons for waiting for EMS to splint the injured parts are:

- A young child in pain cannot be relied on to be cooperative.
- Someone who has only first aid training can apply splints incorrectly. A splint that is applied too tightly or positions a limb incorrectly can restrict circulation and cause further pain and damage.
- EMS providers have received training on how to apply a splint easily and safely.
- Unnecessary movement of the injury during splinting can cause additional pain and damage to the bone, soft tissue, blood vessels, and nerves.
- Usually, a child will splint an injured body part by not moving it to avoid pain.

First Aid Tip

Splinting
It is generally better to wait for EMS to arrive to splint an injured body part. You may need to splint the injured body part to control bleeding or if you must move the child. To splint an injured body part, you can:

- Put it against an uninjured part of the child's body. For example, you can tape an injured finger to an uninjured finger next to it (commonly called, "buddy-splinting").
- Use a rigid object that is big enough to cross the joint above and below the injury. Put the rigid object against the injured body part and use cloth or tape to hold it in place. This helps to prevent the broken bone edges from moving.

If a wound is present follow Standard Precautions. To control bleeding when there may be a bone injury, apply pressure on the tissues above or below the injury or directly on any bone end that is bleeding. Be sure that the ends of the broken bone do not move during the application of pressure to control bleeding. If the bone ends move, further injury might occur. If you need to control bleeding, **splinting** the injured area may help to prevent movement at the site of the injury.

After controlling bleeding, cover the wound with a sterile dressing or a large, clean cloth to keep the injured area as clean as possible.

Apply ice or cold packs wrapped in a thin towel to reduce swelling and pain. Elevate a splinted injured arm or leg, as long as it does not cause increased pain. This also helps to reduce swelling and pain. Do not move anyone you suspect might have a neck or spinal injury.

First Aid Tip

- Do not attempt to clean an open wound if you suspect that there is a fracture.
- Do not give the child who might have a broken bone anything to eat or drink.
- Do not move anyone you suspect might have a neck or spinal injury.

Injuries to the Spine

What Should You Know

The **spinal cord** is the bony column that surrounds and protects the nerves of the spine. A **spinal injury** is an injury that damages the spinal cord. These nerves of the spine allow sensation and movement throughout the body. Any serious injury to the spinal cord and nerves can cause **paralysis** below the area of injury. Paralysis is a permanent loss of feeling and movement.

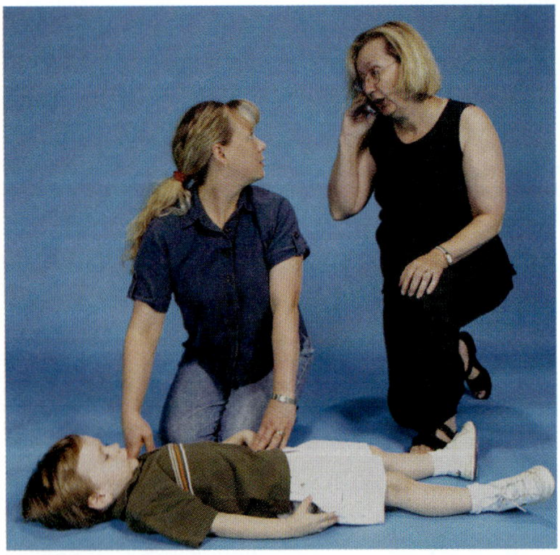

Figure 5-4

Keep a child with a suspected back or neck (spinal) injury still. A child who is unresponsive after an injury should be treated as if there may be a spinal injury.

Fractures of the spine are uncommon in children. However, any child who is unresponsive after an event that could have caused a spinal injury should be treated as if he has a spinal injury (**Figure 5-4**). If a child with a spinal injury is allowed to sit up or is improperly handled, nerves can become damaged which can cause paralysis and death.

Did You Know?

Sports-Related Injuries

Children as young as 4 years of age participate in organized individual and team sports. Around 4 million children seek treatment in hospital emergency rooms every year as a result of sports-related injuries, and about another 8 million are treated by health professionals for these injuries. Follow these guidelines to help prevent an injury:

- The coach should have experience, training, and education in the health risks of training children too vigorously.
- All coaches, whether paid or volunteer, should have first aid skills.
- Children should have a complete physical examination before participating in sports.
- Children should know what safety equipment is necessary, and they should use it consistently. Equipment should fit properly.
- Playing areas should be free of hazardous debris.
- Warm-up and cool-down activities should always take place.
- Pain is an indication that something is wrong. Children should never be told to "work through it."

Adapted from: "Sports and Injuries", The National Youth Sports Foundation for the Prevention of Athletic Injuries, Inc.

What You Should Look For

- Loss of responsiveness.
- Child is unable to walk or experiences muscle spasms.
- Neck or back pain.
- Localized tenderness, swelling, or bruising.
- Headaches—child complains of pain radiating through shoulders.
- Child is unable to move arms or legs.
- Loss of mobility—child will not want to move the neck.

What You Should Do

First Aid Care for Spinal Injuries

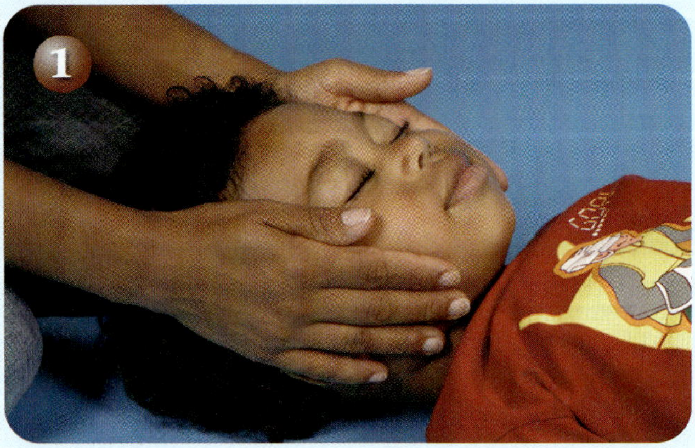

1. Ensure that the child does not move and that nobody moves him. Do not struggle with the child or hold him down. A child with a spine injury will either be unable to move or will find that moving hurts and will not want to move.

2. Call EMS to transport the child to a medical facility.

Algorithm

First Aid for Bone, Joint, and Muscle Injuries

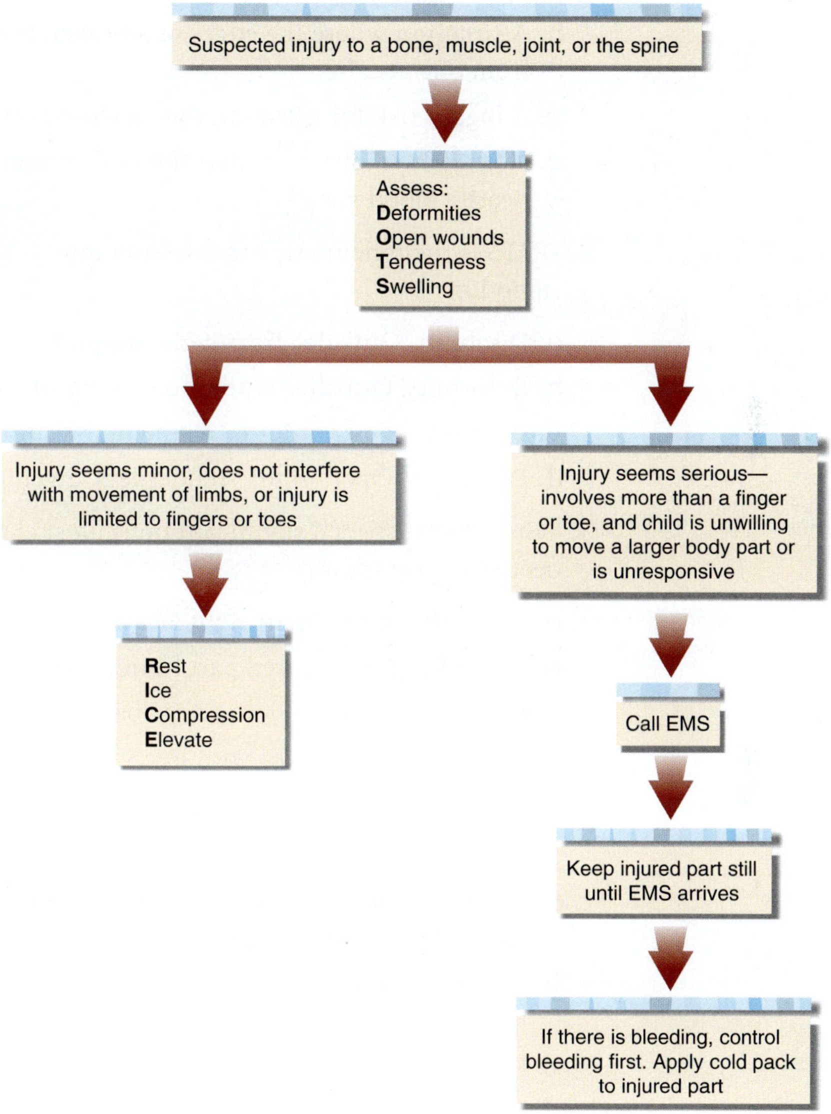

Check Your Knowledge

1. An open fracture is:
   - **a.** Easier to manage than a closed fracture.
   - **b.** A situation where the edges of a broken bone separate from one another.
   - **c.** A bigger risk for infection than a closed fracture.
   - **d.** Not likely to bleed because the broken bone presses on nearby blood vessels.
2. DOTS is the mnemonic for assessing injury. The letters stand for:
   - **a.** Disability, Outside, Treatment, Support.
   - **b.** Deformity, Outside, Tenderness, Support.
   - **c.** Deformity, Open injury, Treatment, Swelling.
   - **d.** Deformity, Open injury, Tenderness, Swelling.
3. When you suspect a significant musculoskeletal injury has occurred, you should:
   - **a.** Splint the injured part right away.
   - **b.** Try to keep the injured part from moving and call EMS.
   - **c.** Put the injured part into an ice bath.
   - **d.** Wash the injured area with freely flowing water.
4. If the event could have injured the child's neck or back, you should:
   - **a.** Avoid moving the child at all, and keep the neck and back aligned as you find the child.
   - **b.** Straighten out any awkward position the child seems to have assumed so that the neck and back look straight.
   - **c.** Push back on the forehead to open the airway.
   - **d.** Sit the child up to take pressure off the brain.

Terms

Closed fracture	When the skin is not broken where the bone is fractured.
Dislocation	The separation of a bone from a joint.
DOTS	Mnemonic for assessing injury to the musculoskeletal system: Deformity, Open injury, Tenderness, Swelling.
Fracture	A broken bone.
Ligaments	The tissues that hold the joints together.
Musculoskeletal system	Bones, joints and muscles, collectively.
Open fracture	When there is an open wound over the fracture caused either by the bone breaking through the skin or by the skin being torn by the force of whatever caused the break in the bone.
Paralysis	A permanent loss of feeling and movement.
RICE	Mnemonic for first aid care for a musculoskeletal injury: Rest, Ice, Compression, Elevation.
Spinal cord	The bony column that surrounds and protects the nerves of the spine.
Spinal injury	An injury that damages the spinal cord.
Splinting	Holding an injured body part still.
Sprain	Occurs when ligaments are stretched beyond their limits.
Strain	An injury that occurs when a force stretches a muscle or muscles beyond their limits.

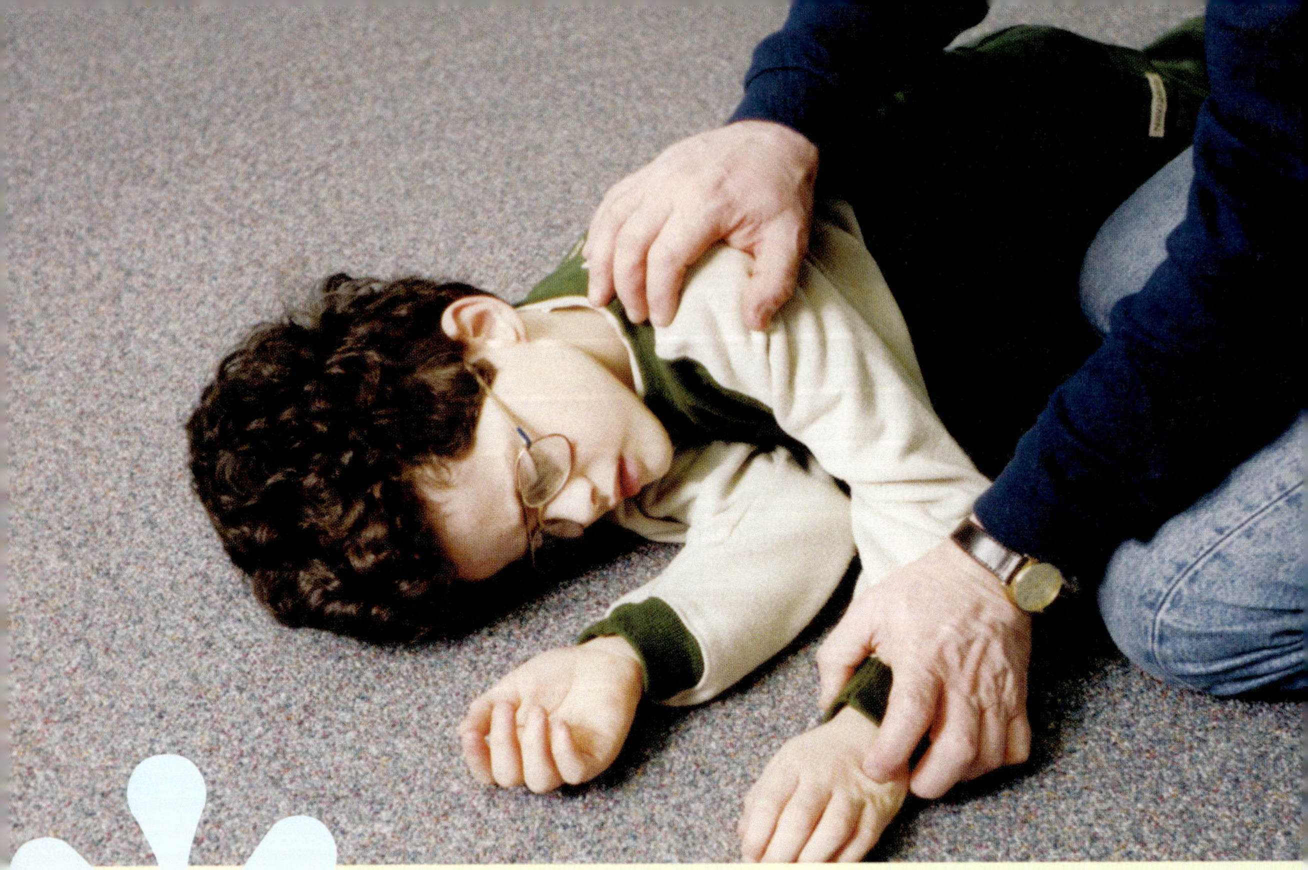

Learning Objectives

The participant will be able to:

- Recognize the causes, signs, and symptoms of fainting.
- Describe first aid for fainting.
- Identify some causes of loss of consciousness.
- Identify the difference between hypoglycemia and hyperglycemia.
- Identify some risk factors for head injuries in childhood.
- Describe signs and symptoms of a concussion.
- Identify signs of an internal head injury that would indicate a child needs immediate care by a medical professional.
- Describe first aid for a head injury.

Topic

6 Loss of Consciousness, Fainting, and Head Injuries

Loss of Consciousness, Fainting, and Head Injuries

Introduction

Loss of consciousness can occur for multiple reasons. Injury, low blood sugar, stress, severe allergic reactions, and even breath holding may be associated with loss of consciousness in children. Fainting is a loss of consciousness that is not caused by injury. Children can suffer head injuries as a result of fainting.

Head injuries are common during childhood years. For every 100,000 children under 5 years of age, eighty-two will suffer a traumatic injury each year. Most of these injuries are caused by falls. The relative heaviness of a toddler's head makes head injuries more common (**Figure 6-1**). After falls, the second most common cause of head injury is motor vehicle crashes.

Most head injuries do not injure the brain, but may leave superficial bruising and/or swelling of the skin, or a "**goose egg.**" The size of a bump on the head does not correlate with the severity of the head injury.

The main concern with a head injury is bleeding or swelling inside the skull. This can occur even when the skull itself does not appear to be damaged. Some internal head injuries can be severe enough to cause permanent brain damage or even death.

Figure 6-1

The relative heaviness of a toddler's head makes head injuries more common.

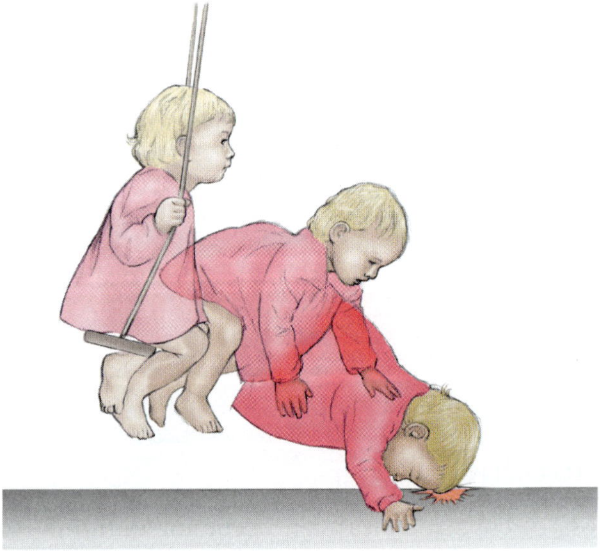

Fainting

What You Should Know

Fainting is a sudden and temporary loss of responsiveness caused by a brief lack of blood and oxygen to the brain. Fainting is not caused by an injury; it is a nervous system reaction to such situations as fear, pain, or strong emotional upset. Occasionally, prolonged standing in a warm environment results in fainting. Typically, fainting is not serious. Usually, children recover from the event in a few minutes without any special care.

Either lowering the head below the heart or raising the feet above the level of the heart can prevent fainting by allowing more blood to flow to the brain. Some children who faint assume an unusual posture while they are unresponsive. These individuals may bend their hands at the wrist and stiffen their legs. Unlike a seizure, there are no jerking movements.

What You Should Look For

- Lightheadedness
- Dizziness
- Nausea
- Pale skin color
- Sweating

What You Should Do

The Eight Steps in Pediatric First Aid:

1 Survey the Scene

Take a brief moment to perform a scene survey to ensure that the scene is safe, to find out who is involved, and to determine what happened.

2 Hands-off ABCs

As you approach the child, perform the hands-off ABCs (Appearance, Breathing, and Circulation) to determine if EMS should be called. It should take 15 to 30 seconds or less.

3 Supervise

Immediately ensure that any other children near the scene are properly supervised.

4 Hands-on ABCDEs

Perform the hands-on ABCDEs (Appearance, Breathing, Circulation, Disability, and Everything else) to determine if EMS should be called and what first aid care is needed.

5 First Aid Care

Provide first aid care appropriate to the injury or illness.

6 Notify

As soon as possible, notify the child's parent(s) or legal guardian(s).

7 Debrief

As soon as possible, talk with the child who received first aid about any concerns he or she may have, and talk with other children who witnessed the injury and first aid procedures.

8 Document

Complete an incident report form.

What You Should Do

First Aid Care for Fainting

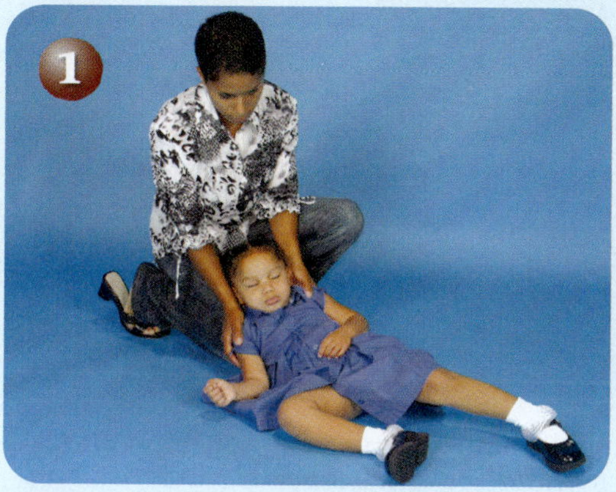

1. Lay the child on her back to prevent falling. If the child has already fainted, position the child on her back and check for breathing. If the child is not breathing, follow the steps outlined on page 34.

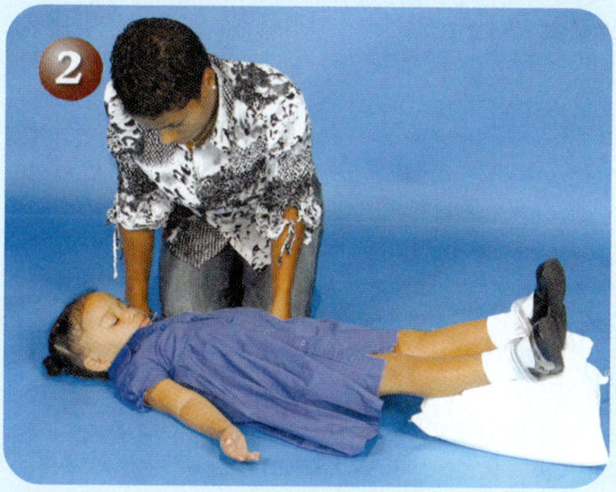

2. Elevate the legs 8 inches to 12 inches to increase blood flow to the brain.

3. Loosen tight-fitting clothing.

First Aid Care for Fainting (cont.)

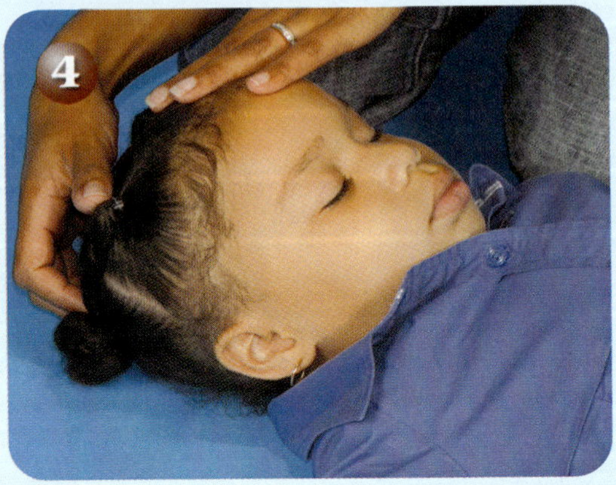

4. Call EMS if the child remains unresponsive for more than a minute or so after positioning her with her legs elevated.

5. Look for a potential cause for the loss of consciousness. Consider the following possibilities:
   - Injury
   - Blood loss
   - Ingestion of a medicine or poison
   - Allergic reaction
   - Extreme temperatures
   - Fatigue
   - Illness
   - Stress
   - Not eating
   - Standing still for long periods
   - A breath holding spell

6. Record details of the event. This includes the amount of time the child was unconscious, possible cause, symptoms and signs (e.g., nausea, vomiting, decreased level of alertness, unresponsiveness, perspiration), nature of any fall, and duration of each symptom.

7. Inform the parent(s) or legal guardian(s) that the child has fainted, as this child may need to be seen by a health care professional.

Did You Know ?

Breath-Holding Spells
Some young children cause themselves to faint by holding their breath. In a young child, frustration, anger, and fear can sometimes lead to breath holding. Often, uncontrolled crying occurs before breath holding. As with other types of fainting, children will lose responsiveness for 20 to 45 seconds. Children begin to breathe normally after fainting and then regain responsiveness. There is no specific treatment other than usual care for fainting. Teachers, caregivers, and parent(s) or legal guardian(s) may attempt to teach the child to manage their feelings to reduce the episodes. However, the problem often disappears as the child matures and learns better coping skills.

Diabetes

What You Should Know

Diabetes is a medical condition which affects millions of people throughout the world. It is a condition in which the body cannot regulate the sugars in the blood stream. This inability to regulate sugar is due to the body's inability to produce insulin or react to insulin.

There are two (2) types of diabetes:

- Type 1 – (previously called "Juvenile Onset Diabetes) Children with Type 1 diabetes do not produce enough insulin to regulate the sugars in the body. These children must take insulin either by injection or through an insulin pump.
- Type II – (previously called "Adult Onset") Type II is the most common form of diabetes. This type is caused by either the body's inability to produce enough insulin or the body is not reacting to it adequately.

It is important to know the difference between hypoglycemia and hyperglycemia when talking about diabetes. **Hypoglycemia** is a condition in which the body does not have enough sugar. Without sugar, the body cannot work effectively as sugar is needed for energy. This condition may occur when the child does not eat enough, takes too much insulin, exercises too much, is overheated, or possibly due to an illness. **Hyperglycemia** is the opposite of hypoglycemia. It occurs when the body has too much sugar in the blood. This condition may be caused by insufficient insulin, overeating, inactivity, illness, stress, or a combination of these factors.

What You Should Look For

Signs of hypoglycemia include:

- Slurred speech
- Drowsiness
- Paleness
- Confusion
- Trembling
- Staggering
- Poor coordination
- Irritability
- Excessive sweating
- Eventual unconsciousness

Signs of hyperglycemia include:

- Extreme thirst
- Drowsiness
- Fruit smell on child's breath
- Rapid breathing
- Warm, dry skin
- Very frequent urination
- Vomiting
- Eventual unconsciousness

What You Should Do

For hypoglycemia, treatment includes giving sugar (granular by teaspoon on the tongue or under the tongue or by drinking orange juice). If the child does not begin to act normally, call EMS and give more sugar. For hyperglycemia, treatment includes calling EMS. If you are unsure which condition the child may be experiencing, either hypoglycemia or hyperglycemia, it is acceptable to give sugar and determine whether or not that helps if the child is awake and aware.

Head Injuries

What You Should Know

Head injuries commonly affect the scalp. The scalp has many blood vessels and even small cuts can cause a lot of bleeding. Swelling can take on the appearance of a goose egg after an injury. These areas of swelling can take days or weeks to heal.

Internal head injury refers to damage to the brain. When the head receives a forceful blow, the brain strikes the inside of the skull, resulting in some degree of injury. In addition, blood and other fluids can accumulate inside the skull, placing pressure on the brain.

Did You Know ?

Young infants have openings in the skull, called **fontanelles.** These areas are commonly known as "soft spots" (**Figure 6-2**). Although the skull bone has not yet formed, a very tough covering of tissue protects the brain under the soft spots. Injury to the brain in the area of the fontanelles is rare, but bulging of the soft spots indicates abnormal pressure in the skull.

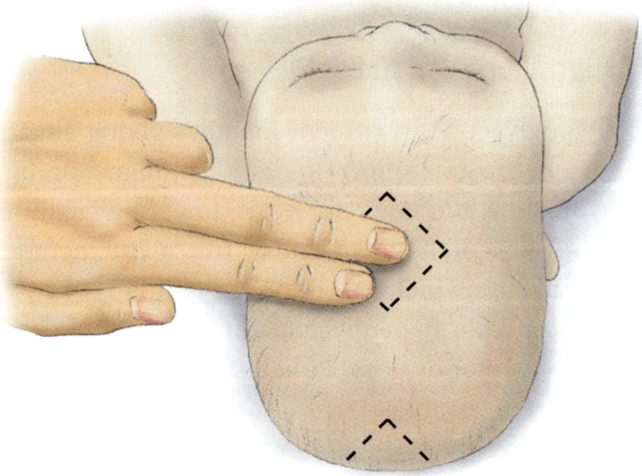

Figure 6-2

Fontanelles.

Concussion is a term that generally refers to the symptoms of dizziness and nausea, with or without a loss of consciousness, after a violent jarring of the brain.

What You Should Look For

- Bleeding from any part of the head
- Loss of consciousness. Appearing stunned for several seconds after a head injury is not the same as being unconscious. Unconsciousness can last for just a few seconds or for as long as several days. Crying immediately after the injury is a good sign.
- Signs of confusion or memory loss. A child should know where she is, and recall the event even if she is upset after the injury.
- Pale, sweaty appearance
- Severe headache
- Nausea or vomiting more than once
- Wetting pants or losing bowel control (when unusual for that child)
- Blurred vision
- Unusual sleepiness, listlessness, or tiring easily

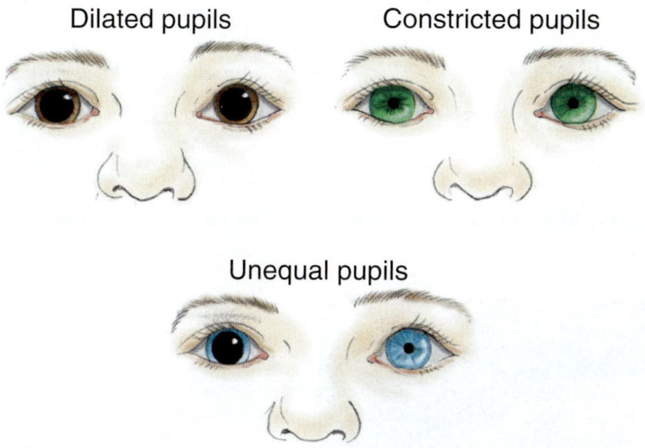

Figure 6-3

Check the child's pupils.

- Agitation, combativeness, irritability, crankiness
- Pupils of unequal size. Check how pupils constrict (get smaller) when exposed to light (**Figure 6-3**).
- Difficulty with walking, speech, or balance
- Seizure
- Swelling of an infant's fontanel
- Fluid (blood or clear) dripping from the nose or ear
- Changes in eating patterns, sleeping patterns, or the way the child is playing or performing (for example, lack of interest in a favorite toy or activity).
- Loss of a new skill, such as speech, walking, or toilet training

Did You Know ?

If the child vomits before regaining full consciousness, you should turn the child's entire body and head together to the left side. Rolling the child to the left side helps to reduce vomiting. Having the child rolled on the side helps avoid choking on the vomit. Rolling the child's entire body and head together (logroll) helps protect the child from the possibility that movement will worsen an injured neck or spine.

What You Should Do

First Aid Care for Internal (or Suspected Internal) Head Injury

1. If a child has a loss of consciousness, treat the child as if there is also a spine injury.

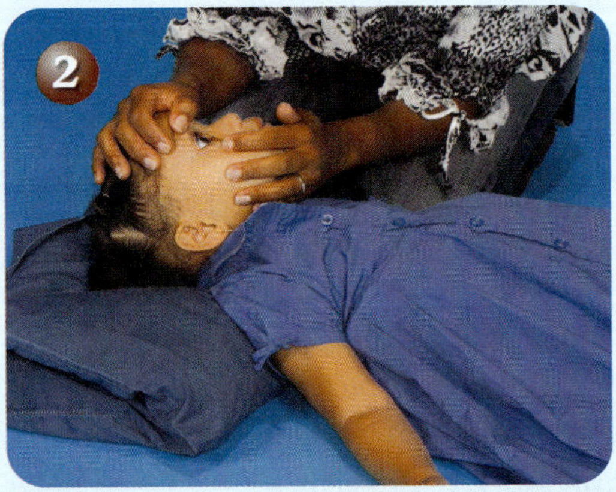

2. If the child is alert, look in the pupils. The pupils widen in darkness and narrow in brighter light. Look to see if the pupils are round, equal to one another, and about the same size as those of other people in the same light.

3. Contact EMS if the child shows any signs or symptoms of internal head injury listed above or if the child lost consciousness.

4. If there are no problems noted on the assessment, the child requires close observation for about 6 hours after the injury and then ongoing observation of any changed behavior for the next few days. The parent(s) or legal guardian(s) should consult a medical professional and become informed about how to watch for signs and symptoms of a brain injury and create a plan of action if abnormalities develop.

What You Should Do

First Aid for an Open Head Injury

1. Follow Standard Precautions.

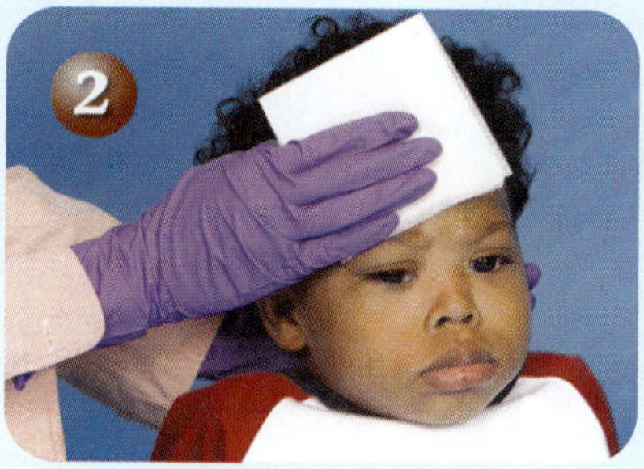

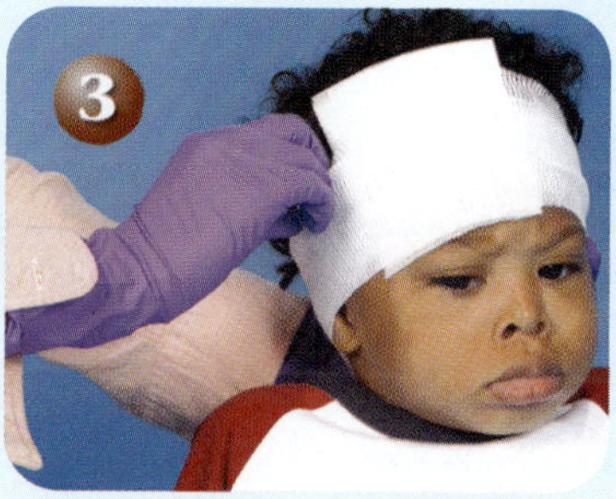

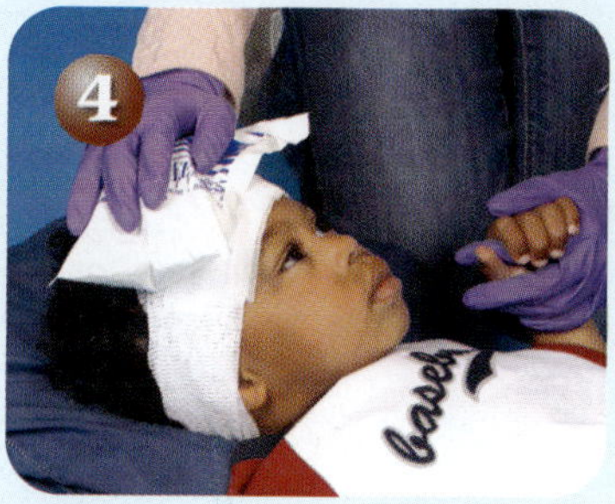

2. Apply gentle pressure to control any bleeding. Gentle pressure is better than heavy pressure if the skull is fractured.

3. Put a clean bandage on the wound once bleeding has stopped. If the bleeding does not stop with continuous pressure, call EMS.

4. Put a cool pack on the injured area for 10 to 15 minutes. (Wrap ice or a frozen object that you are using as a cold pack in a thin cloth so that direct contact with skin does not cause injury.)

First Aid Tip

Sleeping After a Head Injury

- Allow the child to sleep if there are no other signs or symptoms of internal head injury and if it is a normal bed or naptime.
- If the child is acting normally before the regularly scheduled bed or naptime, allow the child to sleep for up to 2 hours without being awakened. After 2 hours of sleeping, when awakening the child, check to see if the child wakes up as easily as usual. Get medical help if the child is not acting normally.
- Note that sleep does not worsen a head injury. The concern is that a sleeping child cannot be observed for changes in behavior or level of consciousness.

Algorithm

First Aid for Fainting

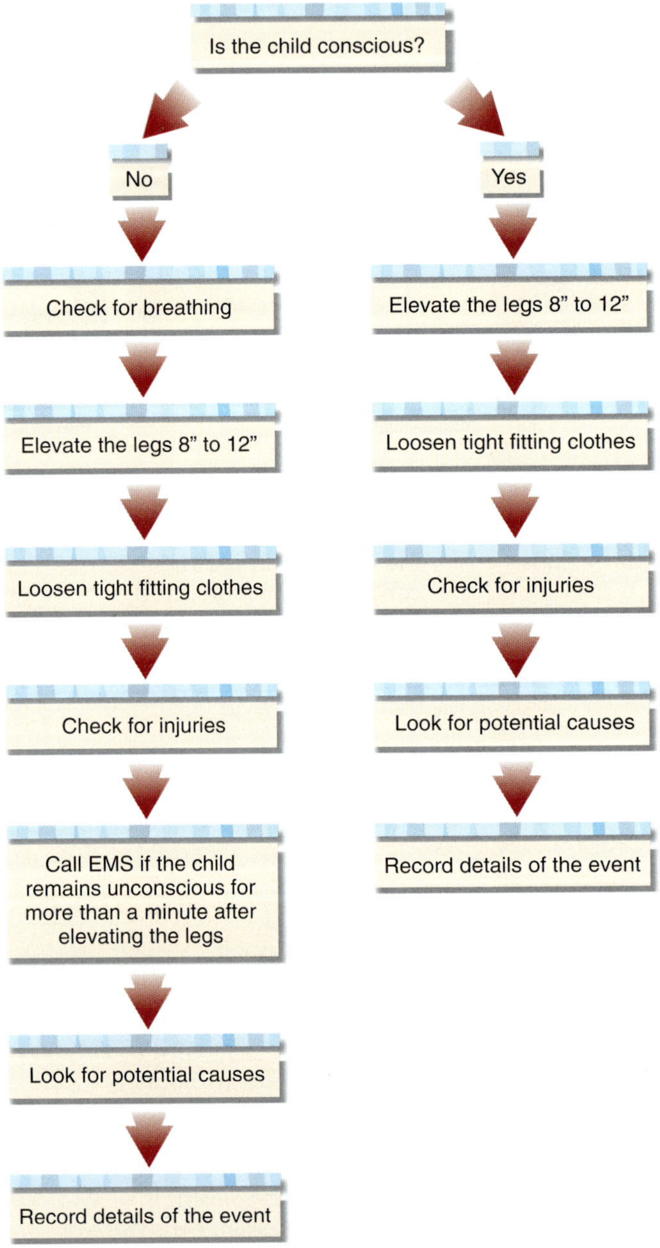

First Aid for Internal Head Injury

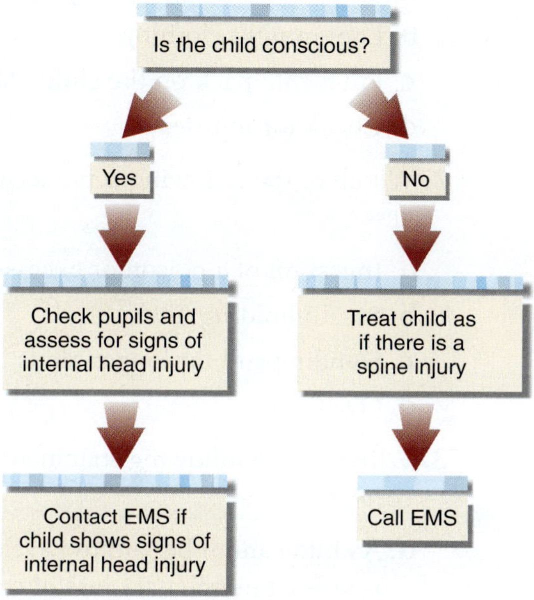

First Aid for Open Head Injuries

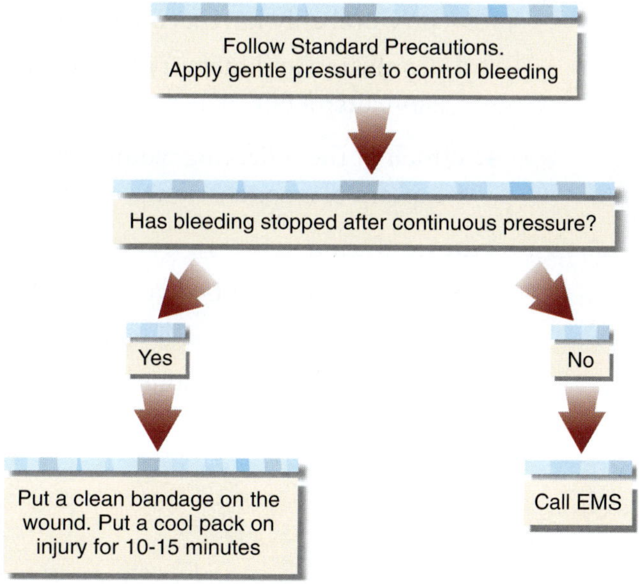

Check Your Knowledge

1. Which of the following is not correct first aid for fainting?
   a. Elevate the child's legs, up to 1 foot above the ground
   b. Loosen tight clothing
   c. Put a cold pack on the child's face
   d. Check for injuries
2. Which of the following is not a cause of loss of consciousness?
   a. Ingestion of a poison or excessive medications
   b. Breath holding
   c. Standing still for long periods
   d. Overeating
3. Which of the following statements about concussions is correct?
   a. A child cannot be said to have a concussion unless there is at least momentary loss of consciousness
   b. A large goose egg bump after a fall is an indication that a child likely has a concussion
   c. Children with a lot of blood in their hair after a head injury probably have a concussion
   d. Confusion and memory loss are symptoms of a concussion after a fall
4. Which of the following would *not* be considered a sign or symptom of a concussion?
   a. Confusion
   b. Amnesia for events that occurred after the head injury
   c. Headache, nausea, and vomiting multiple times
   d. Silence in the first moments after a fall, followed by crying

Terms

Concussion	Generally refers to the symptoms of dizziness and nausea, with or without loss of consciousness, after a violent jarring of the brain.
Diabetes	A disease in which the body is unable to regulate sugar normally because of a deficiency or lack of insulin or an inability to react to insulin.
Fainting	A sudden and temporary loss of consciousness caused by a brief lack of blood and oxygen to the brain.
Fontanelles	Openings in the skull found in young infants, often called soft spots.
Goose egg	Superficial bruising and/or swelling of the skin on the head.
Hyperglycemia	Abnormally high blood sugar level.
Hypoglycemia	Abnormally low blood sugar level.
Internal head injury	Damage to the brain. When the head receives a forceful blow, the brain strikes the inside of the skull, resulting in some degree of injury.

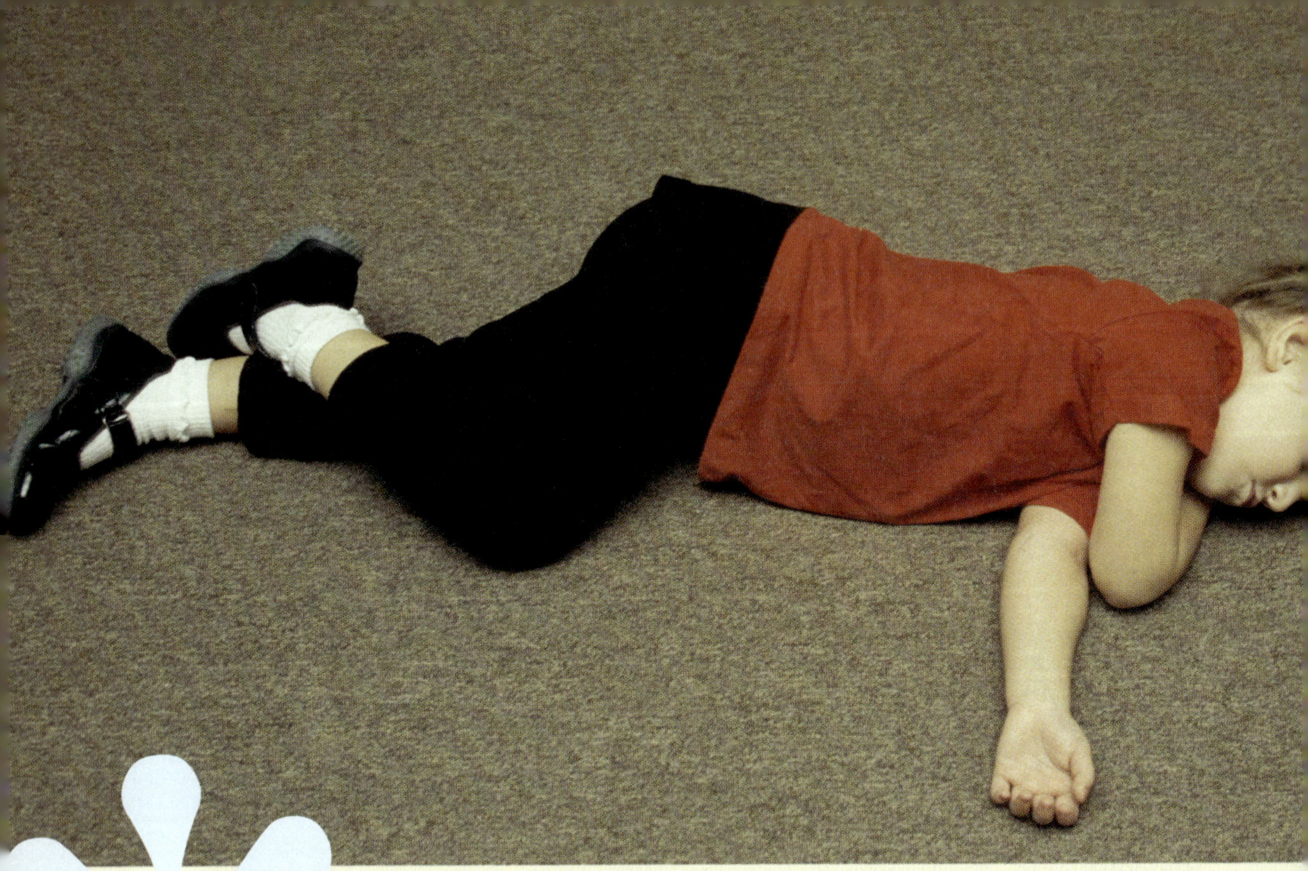

Learning Objectives

The participant will be able to:

- Recognize convulsive and non-convulsive seizures.
- Identify appropriate first aid for convulsive or non-convulsive seizures.

Topic 7

Convulsions and Seizures

Seizures

Introduction

Seizures are caused by a disturbance in the electrical impulses of the brain. These disturbances result in a variety of body responses. These range from the very mild, such as a few moments of staring, to the more severe, such as loss of consciousness and convulsions.

A seizure can be convulsive or non-convulsive. **Convulsive seizures** are characterized by involuntary muscle contractions and body movement. **Non-convulsive seizures** are associated with confusion and loss of awareness.

What You Should Know

A variety of conditions can cause a seizure, including: an inherited disorder, high fever, head injury, serious illness, or poisoning. A child who experiences a seizure for the first time should always receive immediate emergency medical care.

Sometimes a specific cause of the seizure can be identified. More commonly, however, the cause remains unknown. Even without knowing the exact cause, a medical professional can usually treat the child with medication to control the seizures or reduce their frequency.

The most easily recognizable seizure involves the entire body and is called a **grand mal seizure.** When a seizure is about to happen, an older child might know that the seizure is coming by recognizing a brief feeling or sensation that comes on just prior to the beginning of the seizure, known as an **aura.** This is somewhat of an internal warning system, which can be a noise, visual change, funny taste, numbness, or another feeling. Some children experience no aura or do not recognize it so they do not know that the seizure is about to start.

Petit mal seizures are characterized by a brief loss of consciousness. The child suddenly stares off into space for a few seconds and then returns immediately to consciousness.

A **febrile seizure** is a convulsive seizure caused by a rapid rise in body temperature. The body temperature does not have to be very high, but the rate of change in body temperature is fast. In a small percentage of children, a rapid rise in fever can cause a seizure. A febrile seizure is not related to a life-long seizure disorder. This type of seizure usually has no effect on the child's nervous system, development, or brain function. Febrile seizures occur most frequently between 6 months and 6 years of age. A child who has experienced a febrile seizure is more likely to have another one than a child who has never had one. Febrile seizures usually stop in a few minutes, without any special care. A seizure that lasts more than 15 minutes is not likely to be a febrile seizure, and EMS should be contacted.

A child who has a febrile seizure for the first time should be seen by a medical professional as soon as possible. If the child has experienced a febrile seizure, the parent(s) or legal guardian(s) should speak with the child's medical professional to get instructions for how to handle the situation, if it happens again.

What You Should Look For

The signs and symptoms of seizure include one or more of the following:

- Loss of consciousness or responsiveness
- Breathing that stops temporarily
- Rigid body with jerking and shaking movements of the entire body
- Neck and back arching
- Eyes rolling back
- Increased saliva production, causing drooling or foaming at the mouth
- Loss of control of bladder or bowels

What You Should Do

The Eight Steps in Pediatric First Aid:

1 Survey the Scene

Take a brief moment to perform a scene survey to ensure that the scene is safe, to find out who is involved, and to determine what happened.

2 Hands-off ABCs

As you approach the child, perform the hands-off ABCs (Appearance, Breathing, and Circulation) to determine if EMS should be called. It should take 15 to 30 seconds or less.

3 Supervise

Immediately ensure that any other children near the scene are properly supervised.

4 Hands-on ABCDEs

Perform the hands-on ABCDEs (Appearance, Breathing, Circulation, Disability, and Everything else) to determine if EMS should be called and what first aid care is needed.

5 First Aid Care

Provide first aid care appropriate to the injury or illness.

6 Notify

As soon as possible, notify the child's parent(s) or legal guardian(s).

7 Debrief

As soon as possible, talk with the child who received first aid about any concerns he or she may have, and talk with other children who witnessed the injury and first aid procedures.

8 Document

Complete an incident report form.

What You Should Do

First Aid Care for Convulsive Seizures

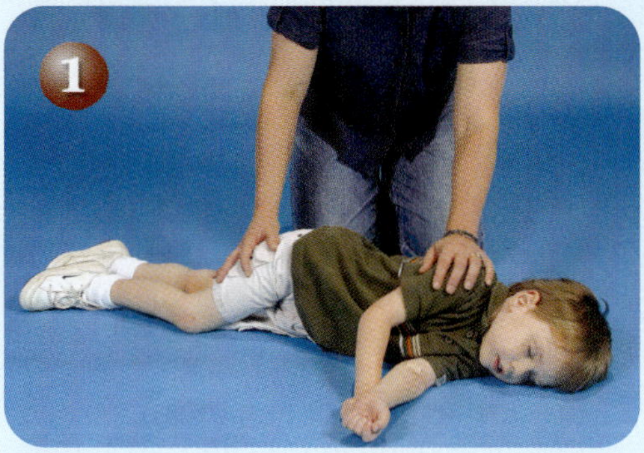

1. Position the child on his side to allow saliva to drain, and to keep the tongue from blocking the airway. Positioning the child on his left side reduces the risk of blocking the airway if vomiting occurs.

2. Loosen any restrictive clothing. Perform rescue breathing if the child is blue or is not breathing.

3. Never put anything into the child's mouth.

4. Move toys and furniture out of the way. Identify another adult to supervise the other children and explain to them that you are helping the child.

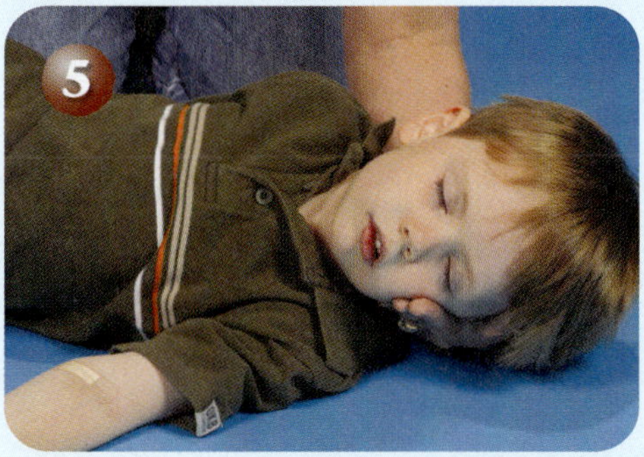

5. Slide the palm of your hand under the child's head to protect the head from injury if possible. You can also protect the child's head with a towel, blanket, or clothing.

6. Note the time the seizure begins and ends and observe the body parts affected. A seizure might seem to last longer than it actually does, especially if you are frightened. Your detailed description of what happened just before, during, and after the seizure is important information to give to the child's medical provider.

7. Call EMS if the child has no seizure history and you do not have other instructions for what to do when this child has a seizure. Always notify the parent(s) or legal guardian(s) when a seizure occurs, even if the child is known to have seizures.

First Aid Care for Convulsive Seizures (cont.)

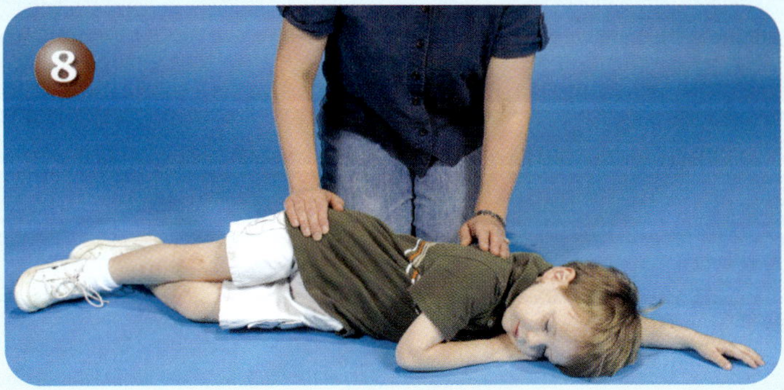

8. Let the child rest, while lying on his side (the recovery position) after the seizure. Recovery from a seizure is usually slow. The child will sleep or be drowsy for a while. Occasionally, children will be overactive following a seizure.

9. If the child who had a seizure has a fever, and you have permission from the child's medical provider and parent(s) or guardian(s) to use a fever-reducing medication (acetaminophen or ibuprofen), give this medication to the child when the child is able to swallow it safely.

10. A child who is known to have seizures should have a care plan for seizures. Follow this plan and call the child's parent(s) or legal guardian(s).

What You Should Do

First Aid Care for Non-Convulsive Seizures

1. Time the seizure and observe the body parts affected if movements occur.

2. Make sure the child is in a place where he will not be injured if he moves during the seizure.

3. Let the child rest if needed.

4. A child who is known to have seizures should have a care plan. Follow this plan and call the child's parent(s) or legal guardian(s).

First Aid Tip

- Do not force anything between the child's teeth.
- Do not restrain the child's movements.
- Protect the child from his environment.
- Do not give anything to eat or drink until the child is fully alert.

Algorithm

First Aid for Seizures

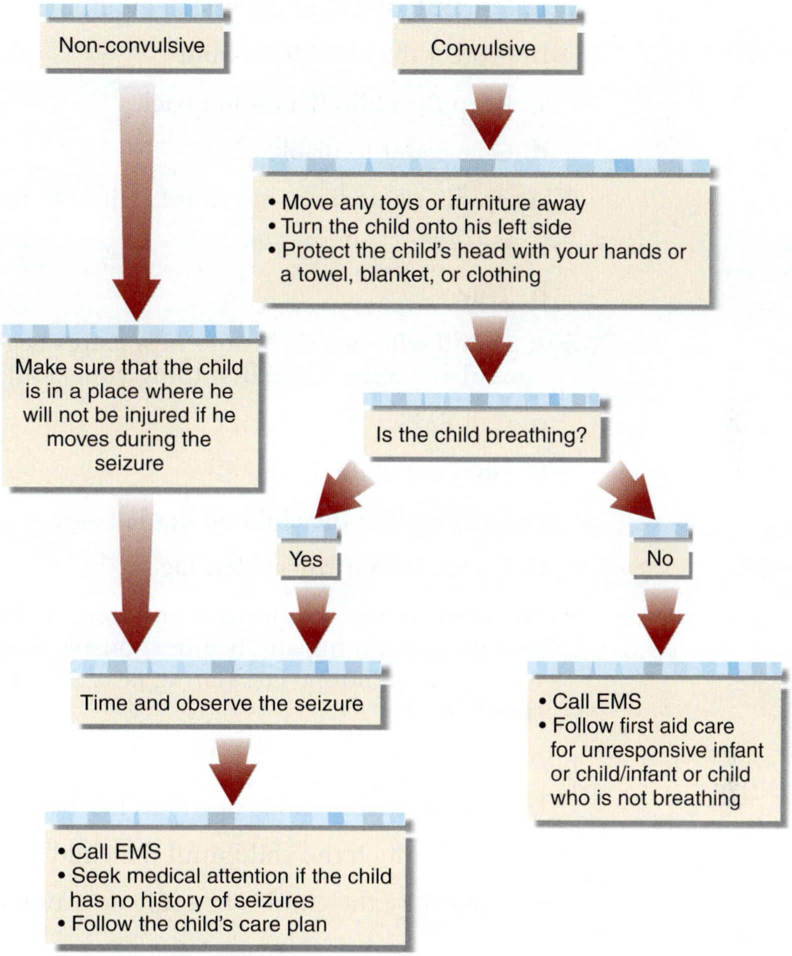

Check Your Knowledge

1. When caring for a child who is experiencing a seizure, you should:
   a. Force an object in the child's mouth.
   b. Protect the child from injury.
   c. Keep the child flat on her back.
   d. Give water to drink.
2. A rapidly rising fever can cause a child to have a seizure.
   a. False
   b. True
3. If a child who has no history of seizures begins to have a convulsive seizure, the first thing you should do is:
   a. Call EMS.
   b. Hold the child down.
   c. Gently place the child on her left side.
   d. Check for a medical alert tag.
4. You are reading to a group of children. A child in the group starts staring and is unresponsive when you attempt to get her attention. The staring lasts 30 seconds. You should first:
   a. Do nothing.
   b. Force the child to lay down on her back.
   c. Gently pinch the child until the child responds.
   d. Make sure the child is in a safe environment.

Terms

Aura A feeling that indicates that a grand mal seizure is about to begin.

Convulsive seizures Seizures characterized by involuntary muscle contractions and body movement.

Febrile seizure Convulsive seizure that is caused by a rapid rise in body temperature.

Grand mal seizure Convulsive seizure that involves the entire body.

Non-convulsive seizures Seizures that are associated with confusion and loss of awareness.

Petit mal seizures Non-convulsive seizures that are characterized by a brief loss of consciousness.

Seizures Disturbances in the electrical impulses of the brain that result in a variety of body responses.

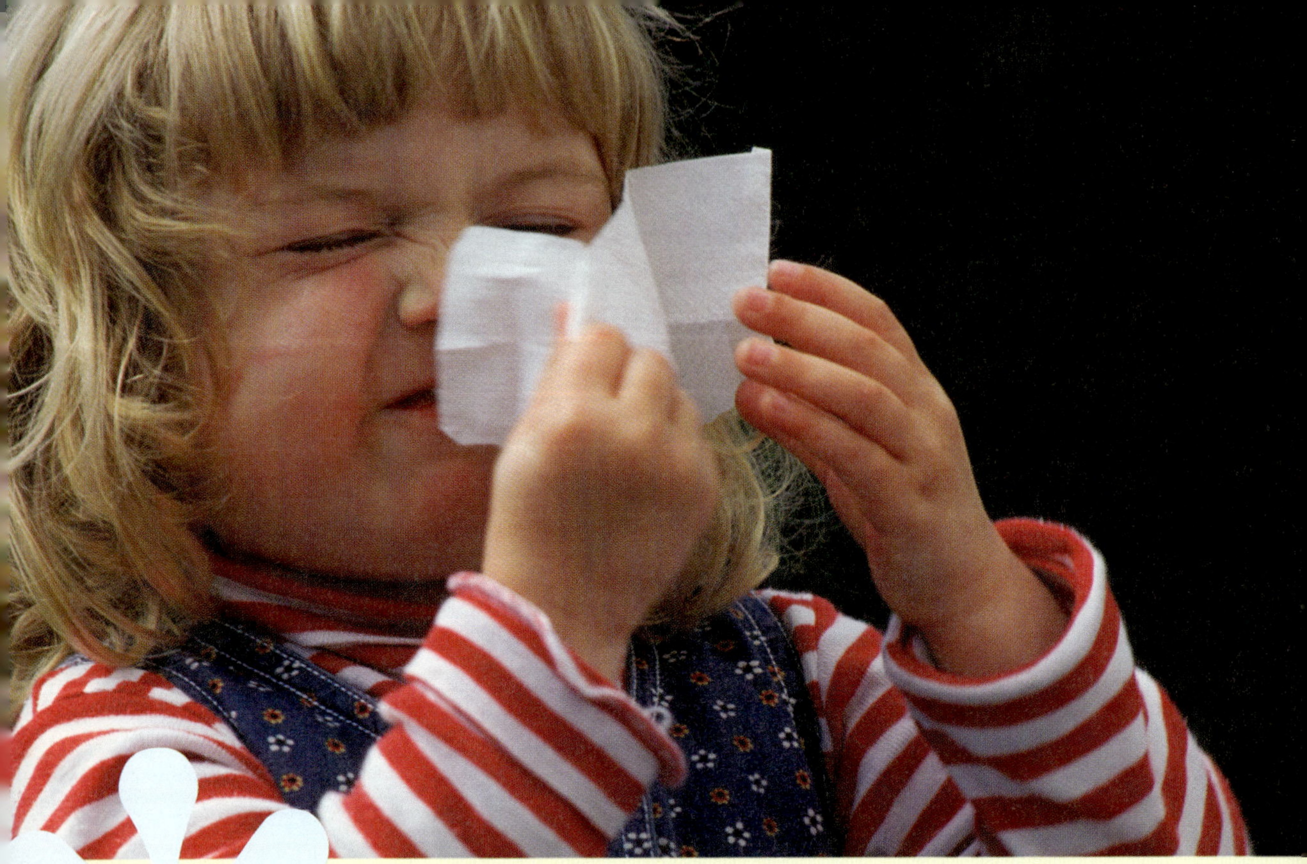

Learning Objectives

The participant will be able to:

- Recognize a child who is having an allergic reaction.
- Identify anaphylactic shock.
- Identify appropriate first aid for a child who is having an allergic reaction.
- Identify appropriate first aid for a child who is experiencing anaphylactic shock.
- Describe the skills required for using an auto-injector (containing epinephrine) for a child who has been prescribed an auto-injector (containing epinephrine) for allergic emergencies.

Topic

8 Allergic Reactions

Allergic Reactions

Introduction

An **allergy** is the body's negative reaction to an allergen. An **allergen** is a substance that the body perceives as dangerous. Some common allergens are molds, dust, animal dander, pollen, foods, medications, cleaning products, and other chemicals. Allergens trigger **allergic reactions.** These reactions are usually characterized by hives or tissue swelling (**Figure 8-1**). Some of the more common symptoms are runny nose, watery eyes, itchy throat, coughing and wheezing, rashes,

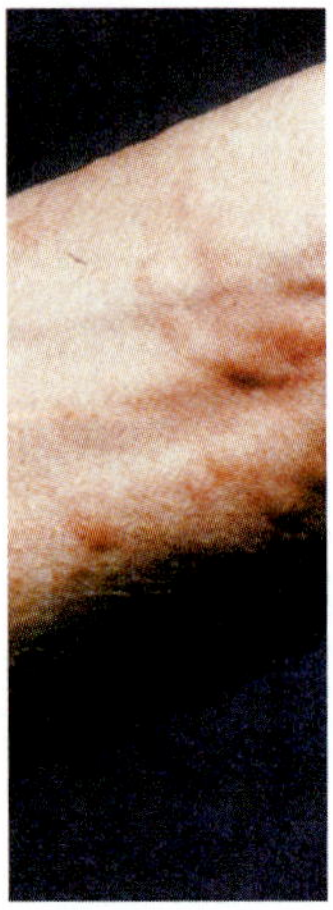

Figure 8-1

An allergic reaction can cause hives.

and hives. Although it is uncommon, allergies can cause **anaphylaxis**, which causes the airway to swell and can be life-threatening.

If a child has known allergies, parent(s) or legal guardian(s) should provide written instructions on potential allergens and what to do if the child has an allergic reaction. Some children will have a prescription for antihistamine or asthma medicine to treat an allergic reaction. Caregivers must know how and when to use these prescribed medications. Medications should be used only for the child for whom it is prescribed and only with both a health professional's instruction and a parent's or legal guardian's consent.

If a child's health professional thinks the child is at risk for anaphylactic reaction, the child's parent or legal guardian should provide an auto-injector of a medication called epinephrine. **Epinephrine** is a hormone that stops the airway from swelling. Epinephrine in an auto-injector is often marketed Epi-Pen and Epi-Pen, Jr (**Figure 8-2**). The auto-injector must be prescribed by a health professional. Caregivers who are expected to use an auto-injector must receive training from a health professional.

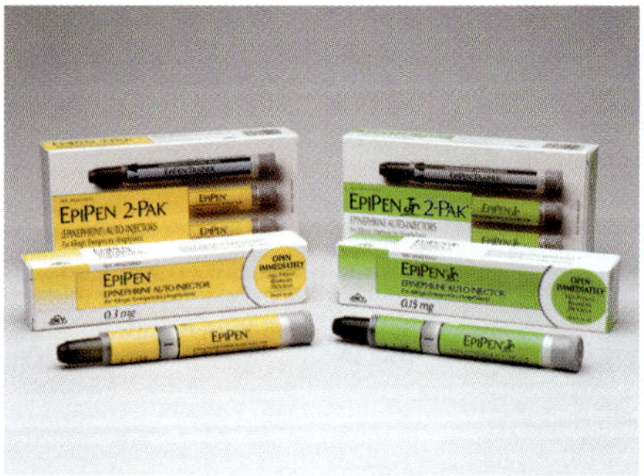

Figure 8-2

Epi-Pen.

Did You Know?

Allergic symptoms may include itchy eyes, runny nose, cough, rash, trouble breathing, vomiting, or diarrhea. The child's health professional may write a prescription for an antihistamine and list the symptoms that indicate when to give this medication. A parent or legal guardian must also sign a permission form. A single dose of prescribed antihistamine upon a phone approval from the child's parent or legal guardian can stop an allergic reaction before it becomes severe.

What You Should Know

Anaphylaxis is a severe allergic reaction and a type of shock that can be fatal if not reversed within minutes. Anaphylaxis occurs suddenly, usually within seconds or minutes after a child comes in contact with the allergen. Anaphylaxis can cause airway swelling that cuts off the child's ability to breathe. If epinephrine is not available, death can occur within minutes.

Anaphylaxis can be unexpected because the child or caregiver may be unaware of the child's extreme allergy to a substance that is harmless to most people. Anaphylaxis is a rare type of allergic reaction. It is more likely to be caused by insect stings or food allergies than by environmental allergens such as molds, dust, animal dander, and pollen.

Anaphylaxis more often occurs in a child who has been exposed at least once, and usually multiple times to one of the following substances:

- Insect stings from bees, wasps, hornets, yellow jackets, and ants
- A medication
- A food, such as shellfish, nuts, eggs, or milk

Usually, anaphylaxis is not the first type of allergic reaction a child will experience when exposed to one of these substances. However, the exposures that trigger an allergic reaction might not be obvious. A child might eat a prepared food without knowing that it contains an allergic ingredient.

Did You Know

An allergy can develop at any time in life, no matter how often a person was previously exposed to the substance.

Did You Know

Shock is a condition that can be caused by numerous factors (dehydration, allergic reactions, loss of blood, infection). The general treatment for shock is to call EMS and keep the child warm and calm. The child should lie down with their feet slightly elevated, unless you suspect a spinal injury. The child who may be experiencing shock should also be covered with a blanket to maintain warmth and attempt to control any further loss of blood. If the child has an Epinephrine auto-injector, it may also be helpful to assist in administering this medication if the shock is related to an allergy.

Did You Know

Common food allergies:

- Chocolate
- Eggs
- Milk
- Nuts
- Peanuts
- Shellfish
- Soybeans
- Wheat

Children who have had an extreme allergic reaction to a specific allergen should have an auto-injector containing epinephrine. Store the auto-injector device at room temperature with the first aid supplies. An auto-injector is not a routine item in first aid kits; it is a prescription drug intended only for the child with allergies in an emergency. The auto-injector is an easy-to-use device that administers the correct dose of epinephrine. The auto-injector must always be close at hand wherever the child goes. If the child goes farther away from the storage place for the auto-injector than nearby rooms in the child care facility, the auto-injector should go with the child. This means caregivers should carry the device out to the playground with the first aid supplies and on field trips.

Did You Know?

In some localities, EMS personnel can give epinephrine shots. In others, the child must wait until reaching the emergency room, unless the caregivers have the prescription epinephrine auto-injector. Find out if your local EMS can give epinephrine and plan accordingly.

Children allergic to certain foods can usually be protected from exposure. Sharing of food must not be allowed. Some child care settings restrict foods that children can bring into the facility and attempt to educate all parents and legal guardians about how to avoid foods that have ingredients harmful to a classmate with allergies. There is some danger in this, however, because it is difficult to educate all of the caregivers who may prepare foods for a child.

Separating a child with allergies from her classmates during snack and meal times may be appropriate in severe cases, but it can make the child feel isolated. Arrange for a member of the staff to supervise a small group that includes one or two friends and the child who has a food allergy when she must be separated from the rest of the children who are eating foods that might pose a hazard. Be aware that some children with allergies are so sensitive that even touching a surface that has been touched by someone eating a food that contains the allergen can trigger an allergic response. The only way to protect such children is to ban the food from the environment of that child altogether.

Did You Know ?

People with allergies should avoid substances that cause allergic symptoms as completely as possible. Check with The Food Allergy Network, (800) 929-4040 for tips on hidden ingredients in foods and for training kits to teach staff about handling food allergies. Also check the Food Allergy Network web site for more tips and information. Read all food labels carefully when children have food allergies. For example, whey and casein are milk products that are added to many types of crackers.

What You Should Look For

Symptoms include:

- Swelling of the face, lips, and throat
- Wheezing/shortness of breath
- Tightness in the chest
- Dizziness
- Blue/gray color around lips
- Nausea and vomiting
- Drooling
- Itchy skin, hives, or other rashes appearing quickly

What You Should Do

The Eight Steps in Pediatric First Aid:

1 Survey the Scene

Take a brief moment to perform a scene survey to ensure that the scene is safe, to find out who is involved, and to determine what happened.

2 Hands-off ABCs

As you approach the child, perform the hands-off ABCs (Appearance, Breathing, and Circulation) to determine if EMS should be called. It should take 15 to 30 seconds or less.

3 Supervise

Immediately ensure that any other children near the scene are properly supervised.

4 Hands-on ABCDEs

Perform the hands-on ABCDEs (Appearance, Breathing, Circulation, Disability, and Everything else) to determine if EMS should be called and what first aid care is needed.

5 First Aid Care

Provide first aid care appropriate to the injury or illness.

6 Notify

As soon as possible, notify the child's parent(s) or legal guardian(s).

7 Debrief

As soon as possible, talk with the child who received first aid about any concerns he or she may have, and talk with other children who witnessed the injury and first aid procedures.

8 Document

Complete an incident report form.

What You Should Do

First Aid Care for Anaphylaxis

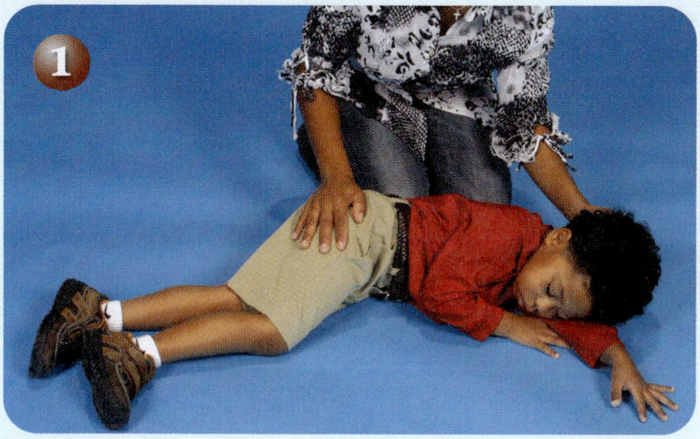

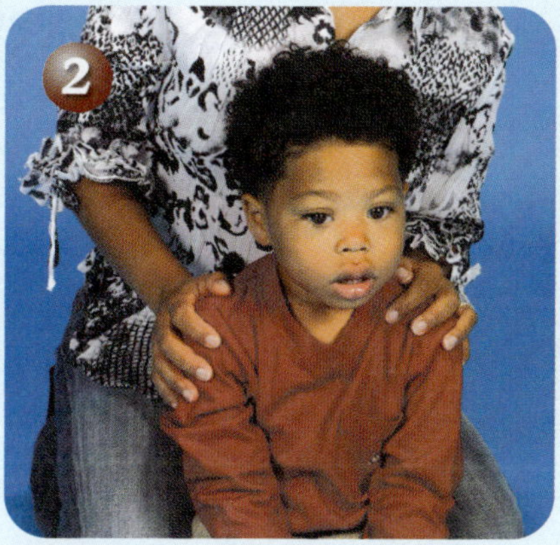

1 Place an unresponsive child on his left side. Check for breathing and call EMS. If the child is not breathing, follow the steps outlined on page 34.

2 Place a conscious child who is having trouble breathing in a sitting position to make breathing easier, and call EMS.

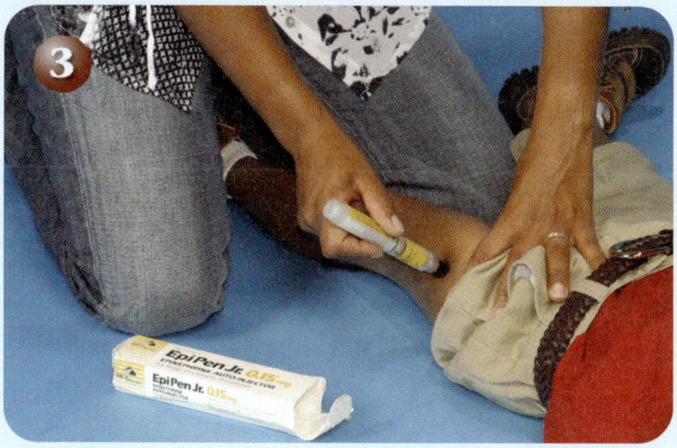

3 If a child has an epinephrine auto-injector, administer it immediately as intended by the manufacturer and according to the instructions of the child's health care provider. A second injection may be needed if EMS does not arrive within 15 minutes of the first injection. If the child does not have an auto-injector, monitor ABCs and treat symptoms accordingly. Administer asthma medication or antihistamine if it is prescribed by the child's health care provider and you have parental consent. Parent(s) or legal guardian(s) should be notified of any allergic reaction.

Did You Know?

- More than one dose of epinephrine may be necessary to reverse anaphylaxis.
- A second dose can be given after 15 minutes if necessary.
- Epinephrine can cause a rapid heart rate, pale skin, and nausea.

Algorithm

First Aid Care for Allergy or Anaphylaxis

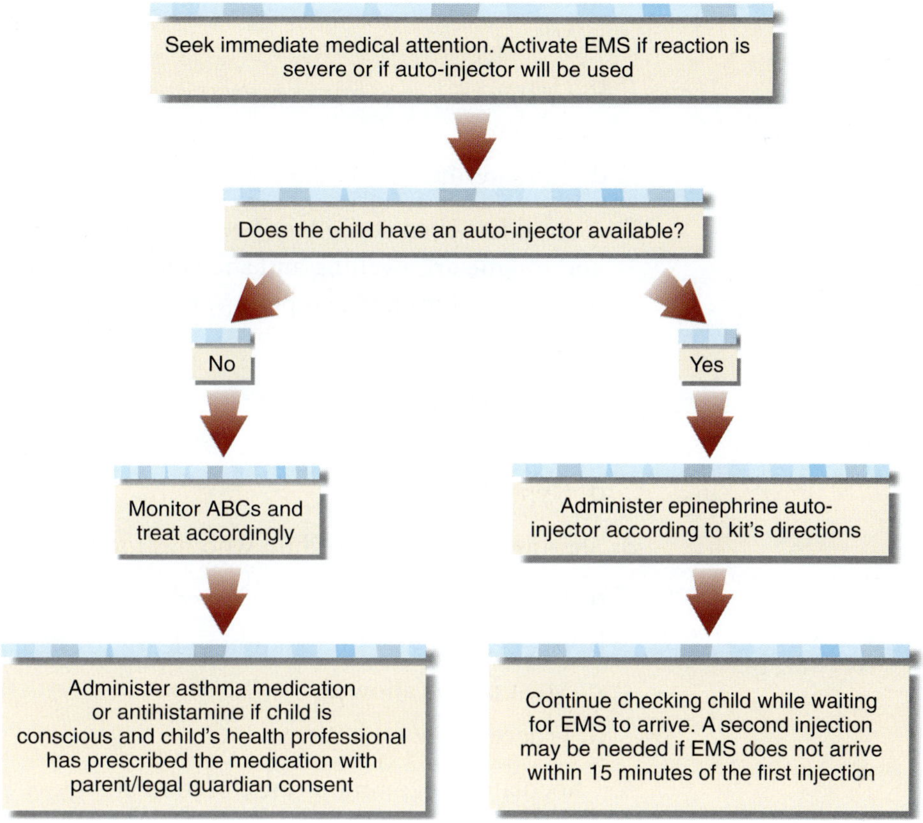

Check Your Knowledge

1. You are checking labels on prepared foods for a snack. A child with a milk allergy should not be given a cracker with:

a. Wheat.

b. Honey.

c. Casein.

d. Corn syrup.

2. A child has been stung by a bee. Within minutes her face and tongue are swelling and she is having difficulty breathing. These signs and symptoms are associated with:

a. Seizures.

b. Anaphylaxis.

c. Asthma.

d. Hypoglycemia.

3. Sharing of food with a child who has food allergies:

a. Is acceptable if the food is baked.

b. Is a healthy way for children to learn to share.

c. Must not be allowed.

d. Is acceptable on holidays.

4. Chocolate is a common cause of food allergy.

a. True

b. False

c. Only in large amounts

d. Only in the summer

Terms

Allergen	A substance that the body perceives as dangerous.
Allergic Reactions	Local or general reactions to an allergen usually characterized by hives or tissue swelling.
Allergy	A hypersensitivity to a substance, causing an abnormal reaction.
Anaphylaxis	A severe allergic reaction and a type of shock that can be fatal if not reversed within minutes.
Epinephrine	A hormone that stops the effects of anaphylaxis.

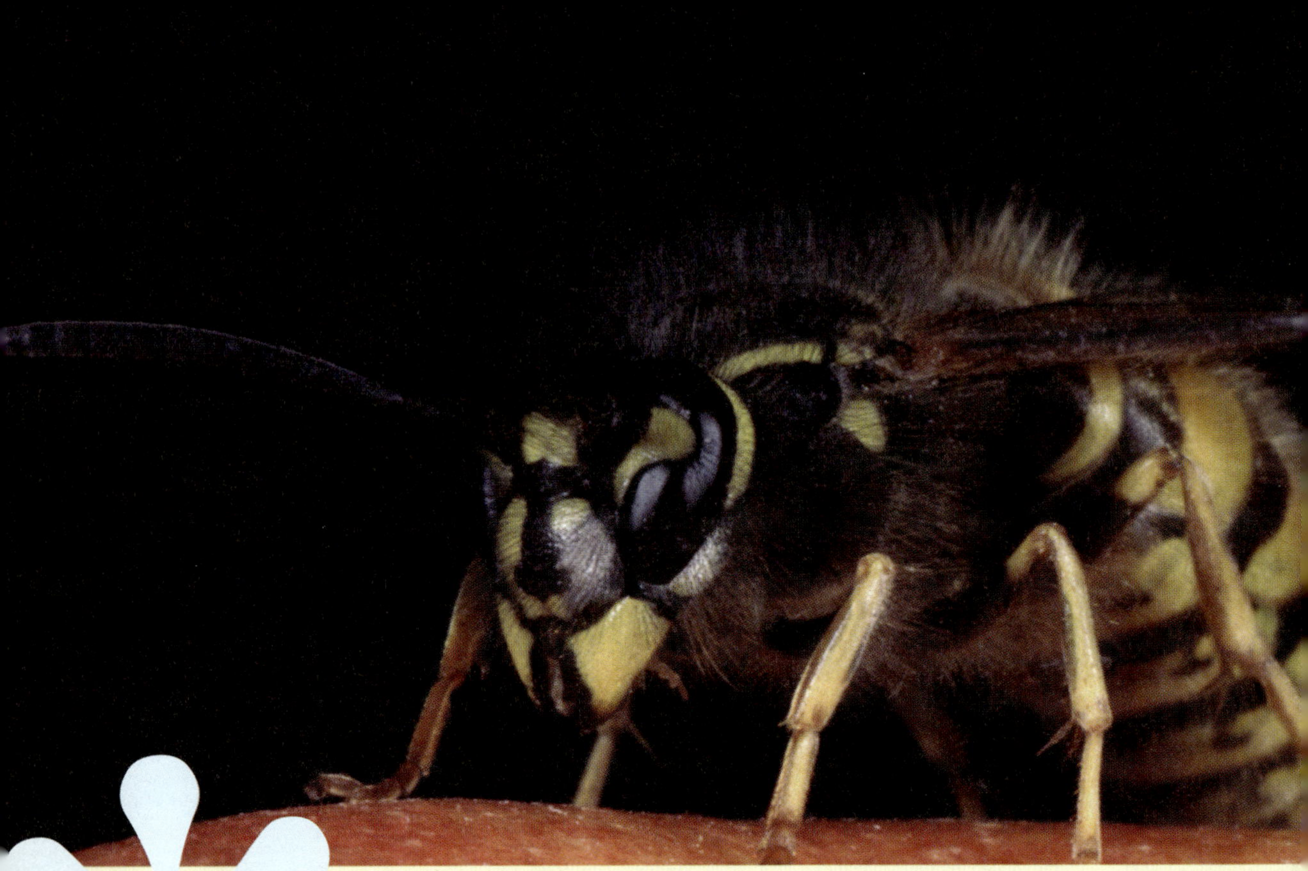

Learning Objectives

The participant will be able to:

- Recognize bites and stings.
- Identify the major risks from human and animal bites.
- Describe first aid for bites and stings.

Topic 9

Bites and Stings

Bites and Stings

Introduction

Animal and human bites are common sources of injury to young children. Many animals and insects that can cause injury are specific to certain geographic locations. For instance, ticks and mosquitoes are common in wet climates, while scorpions are found in dry desert areas. You should know how to provide first aid care for common types of bites or stings in your area. The poison center can advise you about local risks and what to do if a bite or sting occurs. If you have a poisoning emergency, call (800)222-1222. This is the telephone number for every poison center in the United States. For more information, visit the American Association of Poison Control Centers' website.

In general, most bites are more of a nuisance than a serious health problem. However, some bites can be associated with potentially serious diseases. The person giving pediatric first aid should handle bites and stings by providing the care that keeps the situation from getting worse. In some situations, a medical professional needs to evaluate and manage the injured child.

Animal and Human Bites

What You Should Know

According to the American Society for the Protection of Cruelty to Animals (ASPCA), dogs are responsible for almost 90 percent of the animal bites in the United States each year. Their love and loyalty make them popular pets. Unfortunately, each year there are nearly 1.5 million serious dog bites. Cats are less likely to bite than dogs, but like dog bites, cat bites are likely to become infected and may cause a life-threatening situation. Exotic pets, such as ferrets and monkeys and wild animals such as raccoons, chipmunks, and squirrels also bite. The teeth of an animal carry many bacteria. Any animal bite that breaks the skin can become infected and some animals may transmit disease when they bite.

The most dangerous infection that can develop after an animal bite is **rabies**, which is a viral disease. The rabies virus is present in the saliva of an infected animal and is transmitted to a person through a bite or cross contamination with the saliva of the rabid host. This disease affects the brain and the nervous system. Once rabies symptoms develop, the disease is fatal. To ensure that this deadly illness does not develop, a medical professional must evaluate a person who has been bitten or scratched by a wild animal or by a pet that has not received a rabies vaccine. Whenever possible, try to confirm the pet's rabies vaccine status from the pet's owner. Never try to capture or restrain the pet in question.

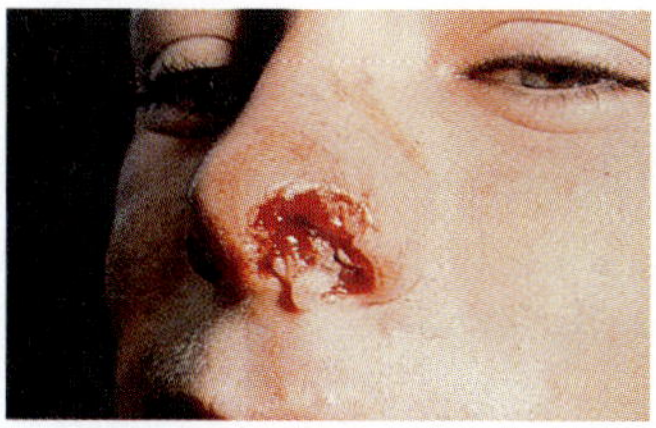

Figure 9-1

Dog bite.

Any warm-blooded animal can carry rabies; however, the animals most commonly infected are raccoons, bats, foxes, and coyotes. A bite from a stray cat or dog is a concern, because these animals probably are not immunized (**Figure 9-1**). Caged animals such as hamsters, gerbils, and guinea pigs are generally healthy and do not typically carry rabies.

Human bites are common in groups of toddlers. Biting is a non-verbal child's way of expressing anger or frustration. Many of these bites are minor and do not break the skin. They cause more of an emotional upset than a physical injury. As with an animal bite, when a human bite breaks the skin, the risk of infection is significant.

What You Should Look For

- Superficial skin breaks with little or no bleeding
- Puncture-type wounds
- Lacerations
- Crushing injuries
- Torn tissues in the area of the bite

What You Should Do

The Eight Steps in Pediatric First Aid:

1 Survey the Scene

Take a brief moment to perform a scene survey to ensure that the scene is safe, to find out who is involved, and to determine what happened.

2 Hands-off ABCs

As you approach the child, perform the hands-off ABCs (Appearance, Breathing, and Circulation) to determine if EMS should be called. It should take 15 to 30 seconds or less.

3 Supervise

Immediately ensure that any other children near the scene are properly supervised.

4 Hands-on ABCDEs

Perform the hands-on ABCDEs (Appearance, Breathing, Circulation, Disability, and Everything else) to determine if EMS should be called and what first aid care is needed.

5 First Aid Care

Provide first aid care appropriate to the injury or illness.

6 Notify

As soon as possible, notify the child's parent(s) or legal guardian(s).

7 Debrief

As soon as possible, talk with the child who received first aid about any concerns he or she may have, and talk with other children who witnessed the injury and first aid procedures.

8 Document

Complete an incident report form.

What You Should Do

First Aid Care for Bites from Dogs, Cats, Other Animals, and Humans

1. Remove the child and others from area. If the bite caused serious injury or uncontrolled bleeding, call EMS. If the child was bitten by a skunk, raccoon, bat, fox, coyote, other mammal, or by any animal that is acting strangely or is not known to be up-to-date with a rabies vaccine, suspect exposure to rabies and call EMS, even if the wound seems minor. The strange behavior may be a sign of rabies.

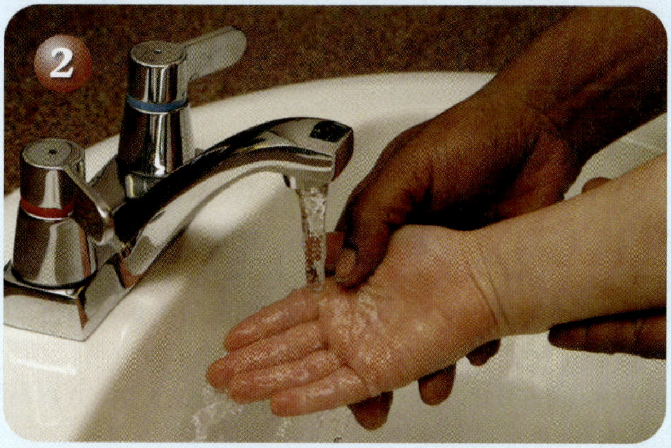

2. Care for any wound or bruised area. Be sure to thoroughly wash with soap and rinse with water any areas where the skin was scratched, punctured, or cut to reduce the risk of infection. If the skin is not broken, clean the area with soap and water, apply a cold pack over a cloth to protect the skin, and comfort the child who was bitten.

3. If a domestic dog or cat bit the child, check with the animal's owner and verify that the animal's immunization for rabies is up-to-date. You should check with your local health department or animal control officer about what to do with an animal that has bitten someone. Unless the animal is known to be up-to-date with the rabies vaccine, the animal will have to be observed for the possibility of rabies. A veterinarian should evaluate any illness in the animal during observation or confinement.

Insect Bites and Stings

What You Should Know

Childhood encounters with bees, wasps, yellow jackets, hornets, and fire ants can be a natural consequence of children's curiosity and exploration (**Figure 9-2A-D**). Also, children may have residue of food on their clothes or hands that attracts insects. In most cases, insect stings do not require medical attention. However, a severe allergic reaction to an insect sting can occur very quickly, without warning, and can be life-threatening. This type of severe allergic reaction that is life-threatening is called anaphylaxis (see Allergic Reactions page 106).

Venomous insects are generally aggressive only when threatened or when their hives or nests are disturbed. Under such conditions, they sting, sometimes in swarms. Children inadvertently may threaten a stinging insect by running into it or playing where the insects are swarming. Symptoms of an insect sting or bite are caused by the injection of venom into the skin. The venom can trigger both irritation and an allergic reaction. The stinger or insect venom may also cause infection.

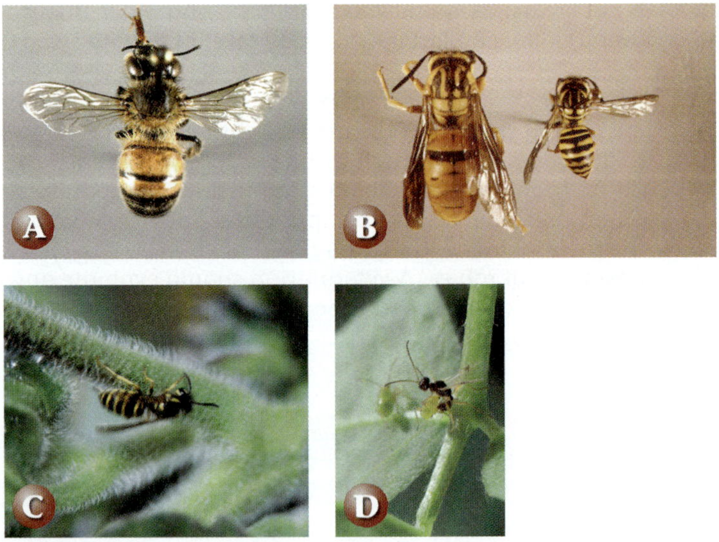

Figure 9-2

A. Honeybee.
B. Yellow jacket.
C. Hornet.
D. Wasp.

Normal reactions to an insect sting include pain, itching, and swelling that disappears in a day or so. Mild allergic reactions include hives and swelling. Although these symptoms could indicate a severe reaction for someone with anaphylaxis or asthma. Severe allergic reactions vary in intensity and usually occur within minutes to several hours after contact with the insect venom. A person who has a severe allergy to an insect sting or bite may have a prescribed auto-injector of epinephrine.

Biting insects include mosquitoes, gnats, chiggers, and some types of flies. In many areas of the country, these insects can transmit diseases that are specific to that area. The insects inject the germs that cause the infection along with their saliva when they puncture the skin. Usually, these insect bites itch and are annoying for a few days, but cause no other problems.

First Aid Tip

Using an Auto-Injector of Epinephrine for Severe Allergic Reactions

- Call EMS
- Do not remove the safety cap until you are ready to use the medication.
- Never put your fingers over the black ejection tip while removing the grey safety cap or after you have administered the medication.
- Do not use the auto-injector if :
  - It is not prescribed to the patient
  - It is discolored (yellow versus clear)
  - Has particles in it
  - It is past the expiration date printed on the side of the box
- Hold the auto-injector in your hand and make a fist around it. Remove the auto-injector's safety cap.
- Place the black tip of the injector directly against the patient's outer thigh (you can inject through clothing). Do not inject the medication into the vein or the buttocks. Inject it into the fleshy outer portion of the thigh.
- With a rapid motion, push the auto-injector firmly against the thigh and hold it in place until all the medication is injected—usually no more than 10 seconds.
- Remove the injector and replace it into its safety tube, and give it to the EMS personnel upon their arrival.
- Massage the injection area after it has been properly administered.

Mosquitoes and gnats are most active around dawn and dusk, as well as when it is humid. Chiggers are microscopic mites that attach to skin with tiny claws and feed on liquids inside human skin cells. They are most likely to attach under tight clothing (e.g., tops of socks, under the elastic band of underwear).

Although many insects can bite, most avoid contact with people. Some insects are attractive to children, even though they would rather be left alone. For example, children love to handle caterpillars although many caterpillars can cause a rash.

Local health authorities can advise you about the types of disease risks from biting insects that are of concern in your area. Ask the local health department or a medical professional in your community about what to watch for and safe ways to reduce the risk of insect bites for children.

What You Should Look For

- Painful or itchy area where the insect stung or bit the child
- Redness and swelling in the area of the sting or bite
- Child feeling or acting ill
- Signs of an allergic reaction, such as:
  - Hives, extensive swelling, or spreading rash
  - Difficulty breathing
  - A dry, hacking cough, wheezing, or tightness in nose, throat, or chest
  - Itchy eyes
  - Swelling of lips, eyes, or throat
  - Weakness or dizziness
  - Rapid heartbeat
  - Nausea/vomiting

What You Should Do

First Aid Care for Mild to Moderate Reactions to Insect Stings and Bites

1. Move the child to a safe area to avoid more stings or bites.

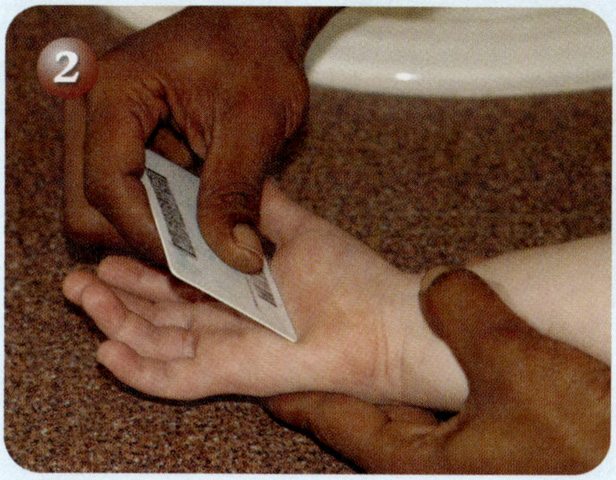

2. Remove any body parts of the stinging or biting insect. Look for and quickly remove any stinger by scraping it with a credit card or fingernail. If the child has touched a caterpillar that left any of its spines on the skin, remove the spines with the sticky side of tape.

3. Wash the area with soap and rinse with water.

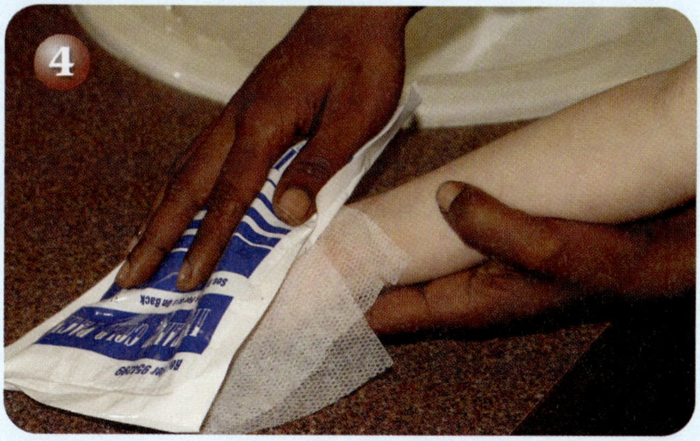

4. Apply a cold pack over a cloth to protect the skin to reduce pain and swelling.

First Aid Care for Mild to Moderate Reactions to Insect Stings and Bites (cont.)

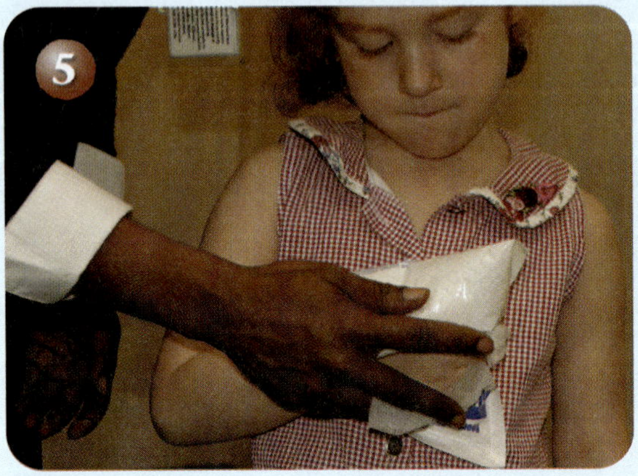

5. Keep the area elevated (above the heart).

6. If the child has an antihistamine or other medication that has been prescribed for insect bites or stings and the parent(s) or legal guardian(s) has given written consent for using it, give the medication right away. If you administered a prescribed auto-injector, contact EMS immediately. (See Allergic Reactions, page 106.)

7. Observe the child for any additional reaction to the bite or sting, and to the medication.

Did You Know ?

Honeybees leave a sack attached to their stinger in the skin. The sack continues to pump venom into the bite site for a few seconds after the sting. Getting it out right away can reduce the amount of venom that irritates the tissues. Yellow jackets and some wasps also leave a stinger in the skin. Since stingers can carry many bacteria; taking stingers out reduces the risk of infection.

Did You Know ?

Avoiding Insect Stings

- Check for nests in locations where children play, such as in old tree stumps, in auto tires that are part of a playground, in holes in the ground, around trash cans, and around rotting wood.
- Have insect nests removed by professional exterminators.
- Children who are allergic to insects should not play outside alone when stinging insects are active.
- Wear shoes and avoid wearing sandals or going barefoot.
- Avoid wearing bright colors and floral patterns on clothing because these can attract insects. White, green, tan, and khaki are the least attractive colors to insects.
- When eating outdoors, avoid foods that attract insects such as: tuna, peanut butter and jelly sandwiches, watermelon, sweetened drinks, frozen sweet treats, and ice cream.
- Avoid being near garbage cans and dumpsters.
- If an insect is near, do not swat at it or run. These actions can trigger an attack. Walk away slowly. If you have disturbed a nest and the insects swarm around you, curl up as tightly as you can to reduce exposed skin, keep your face down and cover your head with your arms.
- A child who is allergic to insects should wear a medical alert necklace or bracelet.

Tick Bites

What You Should Know

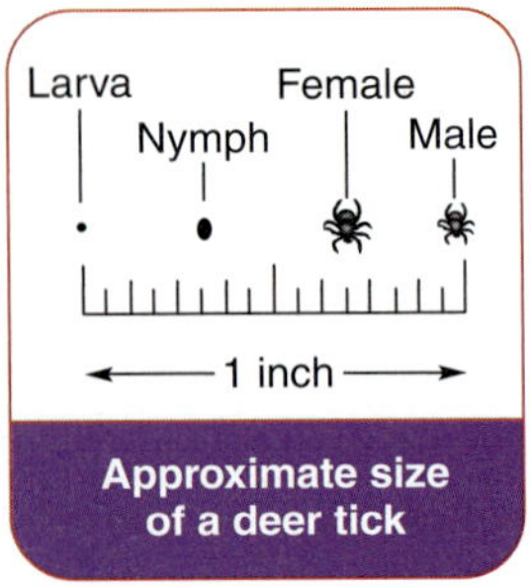

Figure 9-3

Scale of a deer tick.

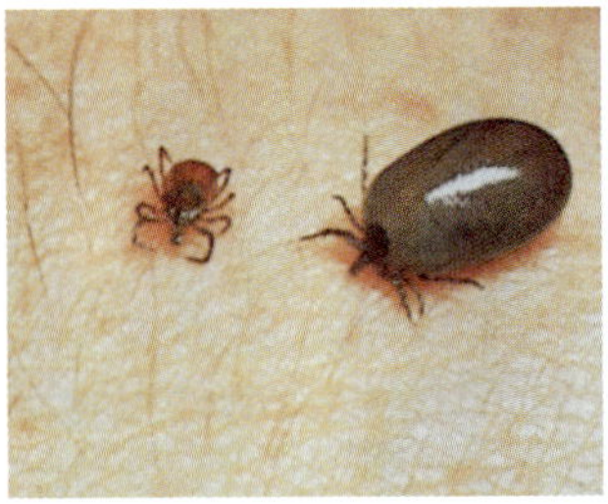

Figure 9-4

A deer tick that is not engorged (filled with blood) and one that is engorged.

A tick is a tiny brown mite that attaches itself to the skin of an animal or human and sucks blood (**Figures 9-3** and **9-4**). Ticks do not fly or jump; they attach themselves to an animal or human who brushes up against them. Diseases carried by ticks include Lyme disease, tularemia, Rocky Mountain spotted fever, Colorado tick fever, and tick paralysis. Many tick bites do not cause disease.

Ticks must feed on blood to survive. It is during these feedings that disease can be transmitted to humans. As the tick feeds, it deposits the waste from its gut in the wound where it is feeding. Infection is less likely to occur if the tick is removed before it has time to feed and fill with blood. The risk of being bitten by an infected tick is greatest in the summer months, especially in May and June, but in some areas ticks can be a year-round threat. Warm weather months are the time of year when children are most active outdoors. The risk of being bitten also depends on the part of the United States, how much time is spent in wooded and tall grassy areas, and the prevention method used. Local health authorities can advise about the risk of tick-borne disease and measures that are appropriate to reduce the risk of tick bites.

What You Should Look For

- An embedded tick or a bump on the skin that is new

What You Should Do

First Aid Care for Tick Bites

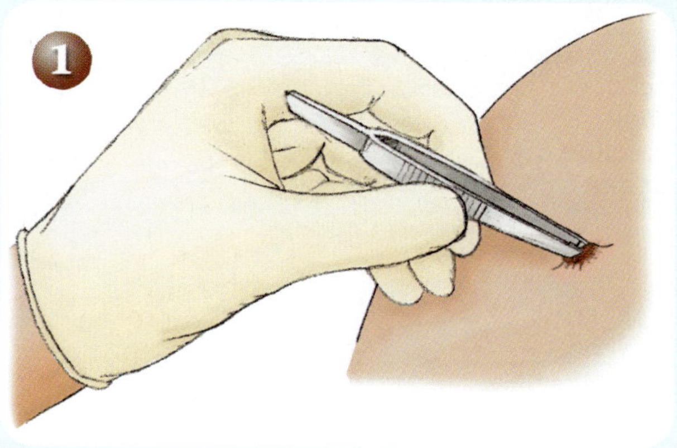

1 Pull an embedded tick out using tweezers.

2 Grasp the tick as close to the skin as possible and lift it in the direction in which the tick appears to have entered, pulling with enough force to "tent" the skin surface. Hold it in that position until the tick lets go. This may take several seconds. Do not twist or jerk the tick, which may result in incomplete removal. Do not grab a tick at the rear of its body. The body of the tick may rupture and the infectious contents may be squeezed into the wound made by the tick's bite.

3 Wash the bite area with warm soap and water.

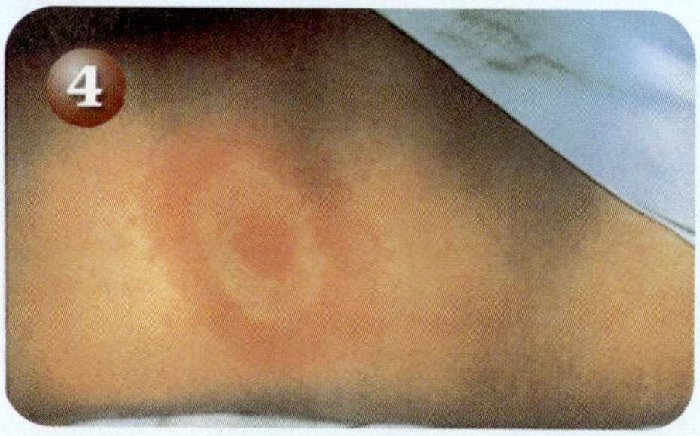

4 For several weeks, watch the bitten area for a rash. If a rash appears, or the child becomes ill, the child's parent(s) or legal guardian(s) should take the child to a medical professional.

5 Inform the parent(s) or legal guardian(s) that you have removed a tick from the child so they are able to watch the child for any reaction that may occur.

First Aid Tip

Do not use any of the following ineffective methods of tick removal:

- Petroleum jelly
- Fingernail polish
- Rubbing alcohol
- Kerosene or gasoline
- A match head that is blown out but is still hot

Snakebites

What You Should Know

Of the 120 snake species in the United States, 20 are venomous. All 48 contiguous states (except Maine) have at least one species of venomous snake; none exist in Hawaii or Alaska (**Figure 9-5**). In some areas snakes may invade playgrounds after heavy rains.

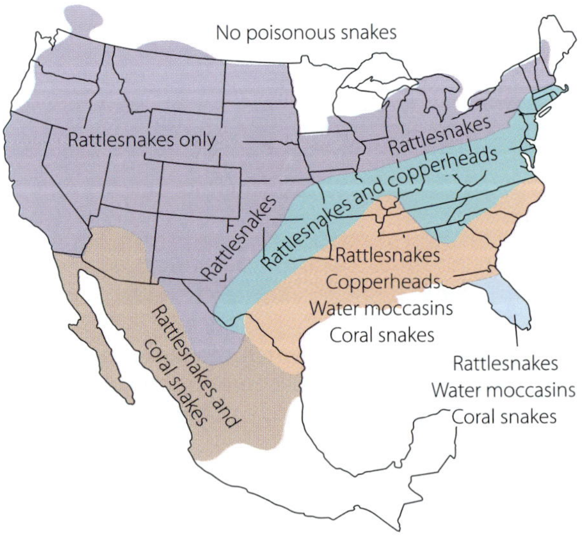

Figure 9-5

Location of venomous snakes.

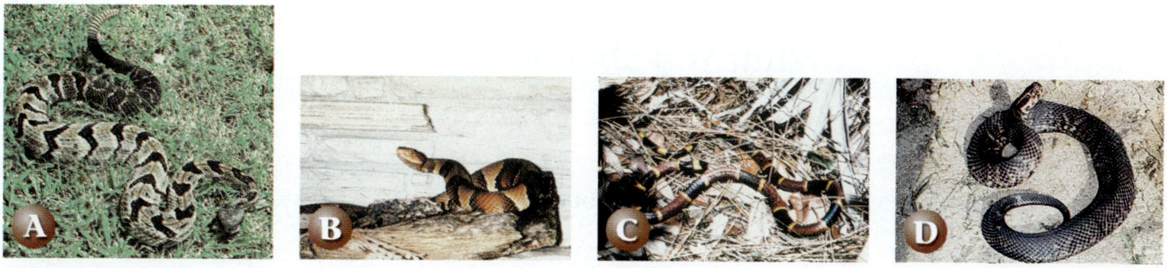

Figure 9-6 A-D

A. Rattlesnake.
B. Copperhead.
C. Coral snake.
D. Cottonmouth water moccasin.

Flooding of snake borrows makes the snakes seek drier ground. Non-venomous snakes can bite, but snakes generally try to avoid people when they can. Although a venomous snakebite is a serious injury, deaths from venomous snakes are unusual. Venomous snakes include rattlesnakes, copperheads, coral snakes, and cottonmouth water moccasins (**Figure 9-6A-D**).

What You Should Look For

- Two small puncture wounds about ½ inch apart (some cases may have only one fang mark)
- Child complaining of severe burning pain at the bite site
- Rapid swelling
- Discoloration and blood-filled blisters (may develop within 6 to 10 hours)
- In severe cases, nausea, vomiting, sweating, and generalized weakness

What You Should Do

First Aid Care for Snakebites

1. Get child and others away from the snake.

2. Keep the child quiet and the body part still to slow the spread of venom. The bitten arm or leg should be kept at or lower than the child's heart to keep the venom from spreading in the body.

3. Call EMS and the poison center (800-222-1222).

First Aid Tip

- Do not use the "cut-and-suck" method to remove venom.
- Do not use mouth suction because the human mouth is filled with bacteria, which increases the chance of wound infection.
- Do not apply a constricting band around an arm or leg since it can cause additional injury.
- Call EMS immediately.

Spider Bites

What You Should Know

Most spiders are venomous. They use their venom to paralyze and kill their prey. About 60 species of spiders in North America are capable of biting humans although only a few species have produced significant poisonings. Death rarely occurs. However, bites from the brown recluse and black widow spiders have been known to cause death.

The body of the female black widow is a dark color with an hourglass shape of red or yellow on the abdomen (**Figure 9-7**). They are found in all 48 contiguous states. Only the female is dangerous as the male is too small to bite through human skin.

The bite itself often goes unnoticed or may be felt as a pinprick. Black widow spider venom is very potent and attacks the muscles in humans. Symptoms are often severe muscle pain and cramping.

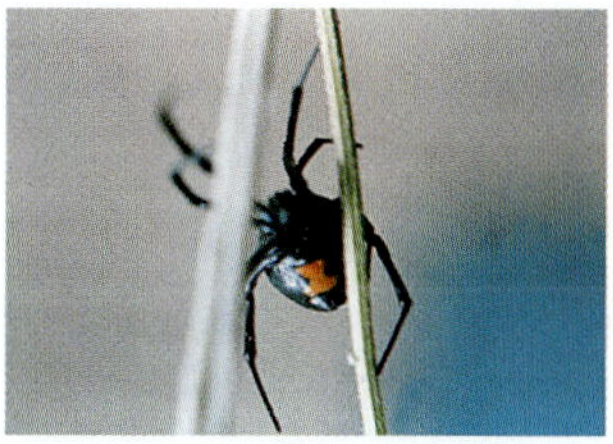

Figure 9-7

Black widow spider.

The brown recluse spider is also known as the fiddle-back or violin spider (**Figure 9-8**). A violin-shaped marking on the back help to identify it. Both the male and female are dangerous.

It is rare to see the offending brown recluse spider because the bite is painless and a large percentage of bites occur while the person is sleeping. Severity of reaction to a bite varies from mild irritation at the bite site to potentially fatal poisoning.

What You Should Look For

- Tiny fang marks
- Pain
  - Pain begins as a dull ache at the bite site
  - Pain spreads to the surrounding muscles
  - Pain moves to the abdomen, back, chest, and legs
- Blister at the bite site
- Mild swelling and lightening of skin color at the site of the bite
- Progressive soft tissue damage

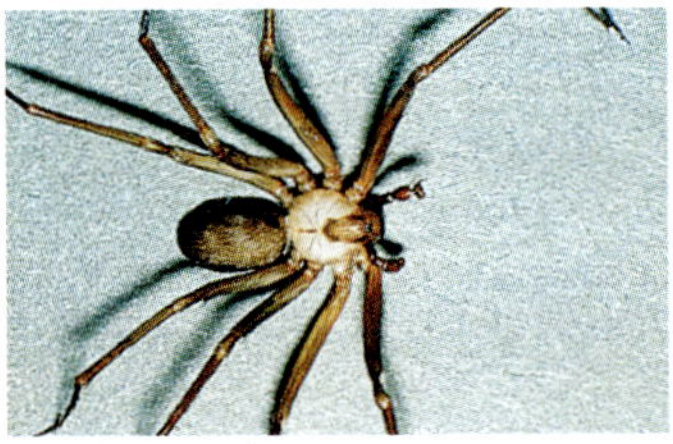

Figure 9-8

Brown recluse spider.

What You Should Do

First Aid Care for Spider Bites

1. If the bite is suspected to be from a brown recluse or black widow spider, call EMS. Wash the bite area with soap and rinse with water.

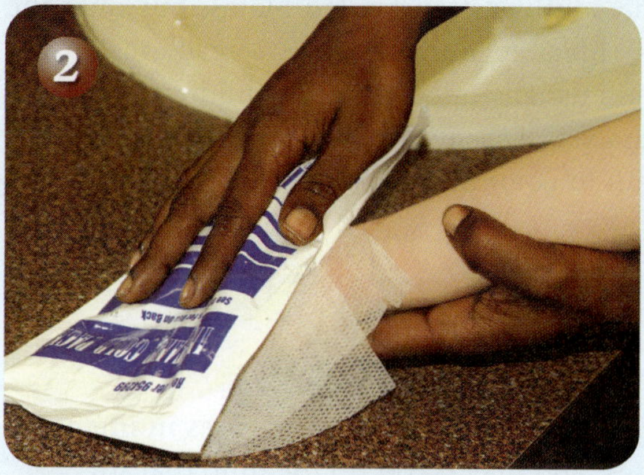

2. Apply an ice pack over a cloth on the bite site to relieve pain and delay the effects of the venom.

3. Call the poison center (800-222-1222) and the parent(s) or legal guardian(s).

Did You Know

For black widow spider bites, an antivenin or antidote exists that is usually reserved for use by young children (under 6 years), the elderly (over 60 years), and victims with severe reactions. Antivenin for brown recluse and other spiders is currently unavailable.

Scorpion Stings

What You Should Know

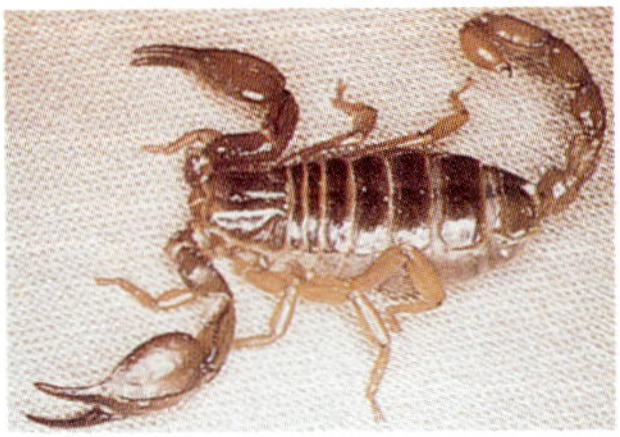

Figure 9-9

Scorpion.

Scorpions look like miniature lobsters, with pincers and a long up-curved tail with a poisonous stinger (**Figure 9-9**). Several species of scorpions live in the southwestern United States, but only the bark scorpion poses a threat to humans. Severe reactions to the sting of the bark scorpion usually only appear in children. These reactions may include paralysis, spasms, or breathing difficulties. The bark scorpion is pale tan in color and is $3/4$ to 1-$1/4$ inches long, not including the tail.

What You Should Look For

- Child complains of localized pain that increases in intensity in several minutes, and may travel up the limb that was stung
- Mild swelling

What You Should Do

First Aid Care for Scorpion Stings

1. Call EMS.

2. Wash the sting site with soap and rinse with water.

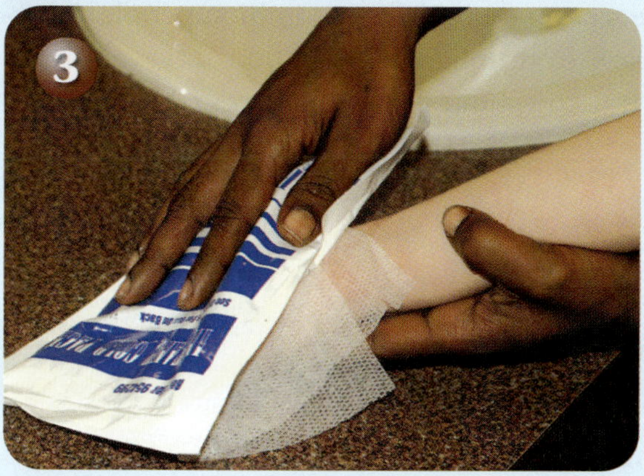

3. Apply an ice pack over a cloth at the sting site to reduce pain.

Marine Animal Stings

What You Should Know

Stings from marine animals lead the list of adverse marine animal encounters. It is important to identify the offending animal, because in many cases care is quite specific.

Each year, jellyfish and Portuguese man-of-war that lie along the shallow ocean waters sting more than one million people. Reactions to being stung vary from mild inflammation to severe reactions. This reaction is due to venom injected by special cells called nematocysts.

What You Should Look For

- Welts with redness
- Burning pain
- Muscle cramping

What You Should Do

First Aid Care for Marine Animal Stings

1. Remove the child from the water.
2. Rinse the skin with sea water.
3. Pour vinegar on the affected area until pain is relieved. Unlike fresh water, vinegar will render the nematocysts inactive.
4. Attempt to remove the loose tentacles by scraping them off with the edge of a sharp, stiff object such as a credit card or forceps. Do not handle tentacles with bare hands.

Algorithm

First Aid Care for Animal Bites

First, remove child and others from area

↓

If the bite has caused serious injury or uncontrollable bleeding, call EMS

↓

If bite was from a skunk, raccoon, bat, fox, coyote, other mammal, or by an animal that is acting strangely, or is not known to have immunizations, call EMS

↓

Care for any wound or bruise, washing and rinsing any opening in the skin thoroughly

↓

If domestic animal, verify immunizations with the owner. Call local health department or animal control officer

---

First Aid Care for Insect Bites and Stings, and Tick Bites

Move the child and any others away from the location where the insects are active

↓

Remove any stinger or body parts of the insect or tick that are attached. Use a credit card or fingernail to scrape out stingers; use tweezers at the attachment of a tick to the skin; use sticky tape to pick up caterpillar spines

↓

Wash any opening in the skin with soap/and rinse with running water

↓

Apply cold and elevate to control pain and swelling in the area of the bite or sting

↓

Give any prescribed medication for children who are known to have allergic reactions

First Aid Care for Snake Bites

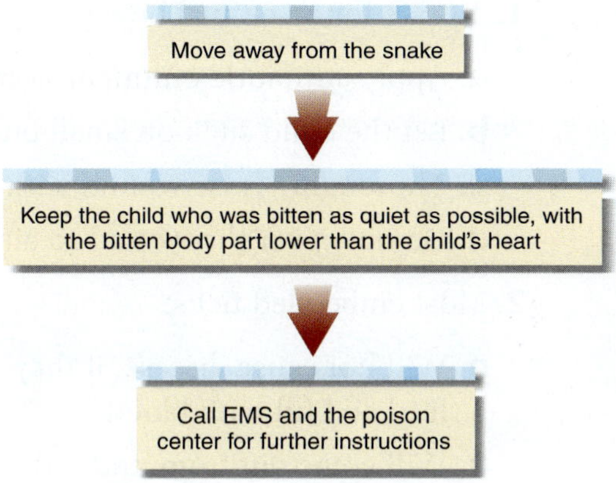

Check Your Knowledge

1. To care for an animal bite:

a. Apply antibiotic ointment over the bite area.

b. Let the child suck on small bite wounds.

c. Thoroughly rinse wound with soap and water.

d. Do not cover the wound so air can dry the wound.

2. Most embedded ticks:

a. Will not cause disease, if they are removed before they feed and fill with blood.

b. Will come out from under the skin if you apply heat to the skin.

c. Occur during the winter months.

d. Do not have to be removed immediately.

3. Which is the best procedure for removing an embedded tick?

a. Apply a layer of petroleum jelly, peanut butter or nail polish over the tick to smother it

b. Apply several drops of rubbing alcohol on the tick to irritate it enough to back out

c. Grasp the tick with tweezers close to the skin and gently pull it out

d. Stick a hot, blown-out match to the tick to cause it to back out of the skin

4. Which is the most important care for a venomous snakebite:

a. Apply a hot compress over the bite area

b. Apply a constriction band to slow the spread of the venom

c. Call EMS

d. Elevate the wound

Terms

Rabies A life-threatening viral disease in warm-blooded mammals that is primarily transferred through bites.

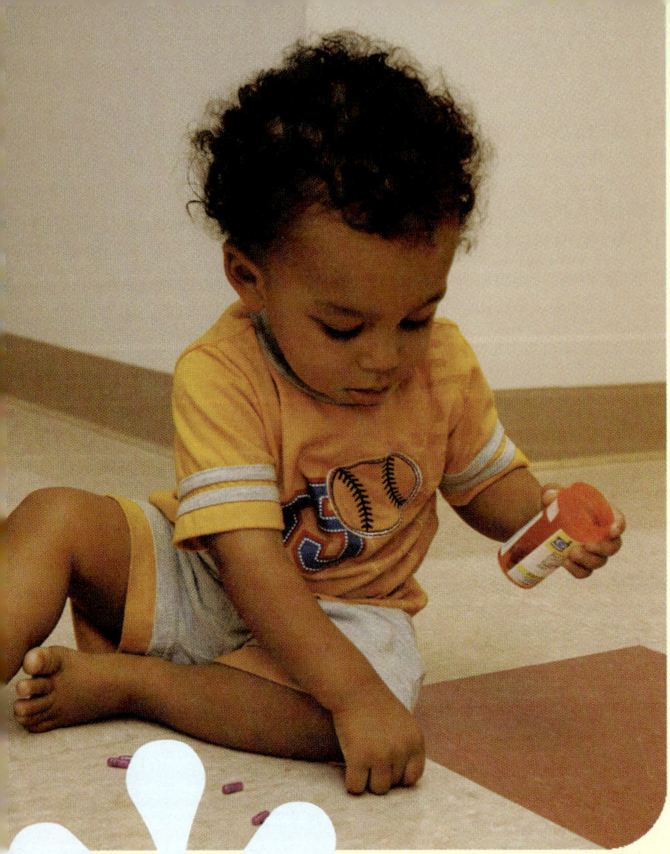

Learning Objectives

The participant will be able to:

- Recognize a child who has swallowed, contacted, or inhaled poison.
- Identify appropriate first aid for a child who has swallowed poison.
- Identify appropriate first aid for a child who has inhaled poison.
- Identify appropriate first aid for a child who has had contact with a poisonous plant(s).

Topic 10 Poisoning

Poisoning

Introduction

A **poison** is a substance that, when swallowed, inhaled, or absorbed through the skin can cause damage to the body, illness, and sometimes death. Often exposure to only a tiny amount of a poisonous substance can have serious consequences. Poisoning is one of the most common causes of injury in children under 5 years of age.

Poison centers, staffed by professionals, are accessible throughout the United States. Currently, the phone number to call for any

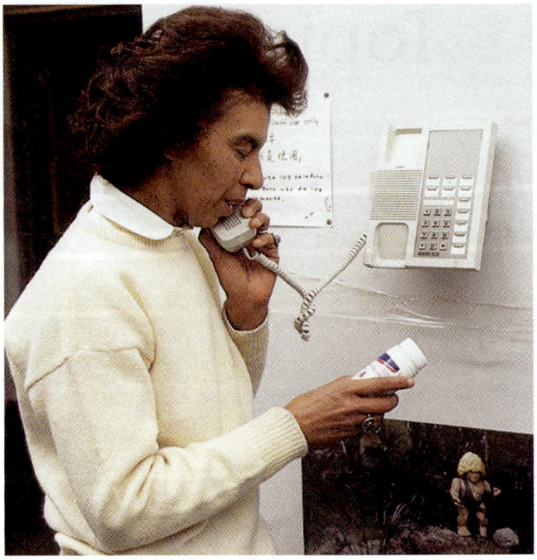

Figure 10-1

800/222-1222 should be displayed by the phone in case of a poisoning emergency.

poison emergency is 800/222-1222. This number should be posted prominently in the child care facility. When calling this number, you will automatically be connected to the poison center in your area (**Figure 10-1**). The poison center staff use a computer database to provide advice, recommend proper treatment, and inform the caller if the child needs to go to the emergency room. Poison centers are also a good source of prevention advice.

What You Should Know

Many products that are used daily are highly toxic and potentially fatal. They can have tragic consequences when swallowed. In general, the poisonous substances that are most devastating to children are medications, cleaning products, pesticides, alcoholic beverages, and petroleum products such as gasoline.

Young children are curious by nature. Colored plastic containers, colorful pills, and never-before-seen-items invite the child to explore. Taste is the first sense toddlers and many preschoolers use when investigating something new, regardless of whether it is a toy, food, chemical, or plant. Poisonings often happen when adults are tired or preoccupied, when children have been left alone (even momentarily), and when proper storage or disposal of a poison is either interrupted or forgotten. Most childhood poisonings can be prevented by safe use and proper storage of household products and medicines. Keep household products and medicines in locked cabinets, on high, secure shelves, or in boxes that are inaccessible to children.

Like many adults, most young children know little about toxic plants. Because children use their senses of touch and taste when investigating something new, it is not unusual for them to touch and mouth leaves, berries, and flowers. Poisonings can occur from swallowing a plant, absorbing a toxin through the skin, or inhaling fumes from a fire that contains a poisonous plant. For the children's safety, learn the names of the plants, trees, and shrubbery around your facility. If a child swallows any part of a plant, take the child and a sample of the plant to the telephone and call the poison center (800/222-1222). The poison control center will advise you what to do.

A small number of plants can cause a chemical and sometimes, an allergic reaction, when they make contact with the skin. The best known are poison ivy, poison oak, and poison sumac, all of which are found throughout the United States (**Figure 10-2**).

Did You Know ?

Child-resistant safety packaging for medication was developed in the 1970s. There is no such thing as "childproof packaging." However, this type of packaging does slow the child's access to the medication so that an adult has a better chance of finding the child first.

Did You Know ?

One of the leading causes of childhood poisoning is acetaminophen. It is a significant cause of liver damage and even death.

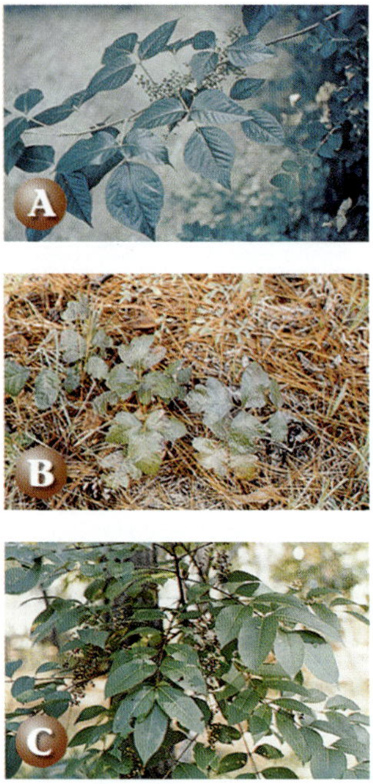

Figure 10-2

Well known plants that cause chemical and sometimes an allergic reaction include: A. poison ivy, B. poison oak, and C. poison sumac.

Exposure to the oil of these plants causes a chemical reaction of irritation and can cause a delayed allergic reaction in the form of a rash that varies in severity (**Figure 10-3**). A child can be exposed to the oil of the plants directly by touching the leaves, stems, or roots, or indirectly by touching tools, clothes, pets, or any other articles touched by the plant. Smoke from a fire containing the burning plant can carry this oil in tiny droplets to the skin and into the nose, throat, and lungs. A reaction can develop from contact with these plants during any season of the year and from handling any part of the plant, not just the leaves.

Poisoning by inhalation can occur as in carbon monoxide poisoning from a faulty furnace, a kerosene space heater, or a car motor running in an enclosed garage. Carbon monoxide poisoning causes rapid unconsciousness, sometimes preceded by a severe headache. It is often fatal. Inhaled poisoning also can occur if a child experiments with intentionally inhaling a chemical, such as the fumes from rubber cement or model glue.

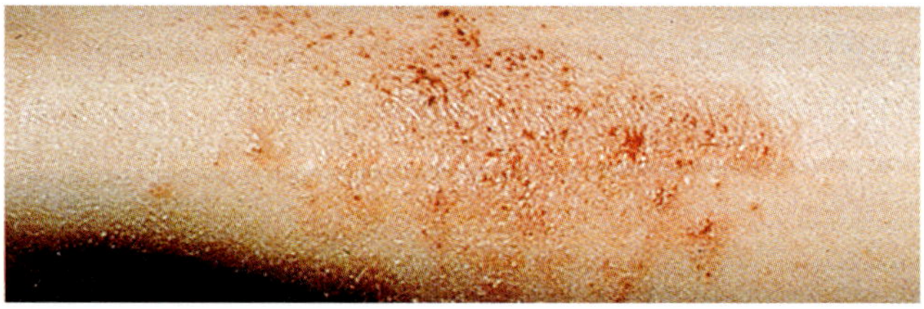

Figure 10-3

Rash from a plant.

What You Should Look For

Swallowed poison:

- Opened container of medicine or chemical
- Unusual odor from mouth or clothes
- Burns in and around the mouth indicating contact with a corrosive chemical
- Nausea or vomiting
- Abdominal pain or diarrhea
- Drowsiness
- Unconsciousness

Poisonous Plant Exposure:

- Rash
- Itching
- Redness
- Blisters
- Swelling

Inhaled Poisons:

- A source of fumes that may or may not have an odor
- Change in behavior
- Change in appearance

Did You Know

In the past, the American Academy of Pediatrics (AAP) promoted keeping syrup of ipecac in the home as a poison treatment. In November 2003, the Academy withdrew this recommendation because studies showed syrup of ipecac was not effective in managing poisonings. Even if children vomit after receiving syrup of ipecac, too much poison can remain in the stomach. While local and state authorities may continue to require ipecac on site, teachers and caregivers should be aware of the change in the AAP policy.

What You Should Do

The Eight Steps of Pediatric First Aid:

1 Survey the Scene

Take a brief moment to perform a scene survey to ensure that the scene is safe, to find out who is involved, and to determine what happened.

2 Hands-off ABCs

As you approach the child, perform the hands-off ABCs (Appearance, Breathing, and Circulation) to determine if EMS should be called. It should take 15 to 30 seconds or less.

3 Supervise

Immediately ensure that any other children near the scene are properly supervised.

4 Hands-on ABCDEs

Perform the hands-on ABCDEs (Appearance, Breathing, Circulation, Disability, and Everything else) to determine if EMS should be called and what first aid care is needed.

5 First Aid Care

Provide first aid care appropriate to the injury or illness.

6 Notify

As soon as possible, notify the child's parent(s) or legal guardian(s).

7 Debrief

As soon as possible, talk with the child who received first aid about any concerns he or she may have, and talk with other children who witnessed the injury and first aid procedures.

8 Document

Complete an incident report form.

What You Should Do

First Aid Care for Swallowed Poisons

1. Gather information and remain calm. Try to determine the following:

   - Age and weight of the child
   - What was swallowed
   - Amount swallowed
   - When it was swallowed
   - The child's condition

2. If the child is responsive, call the poison center (800/222-1222). Have the child and the poison container with you. Follow the instructions you receive from the poison control center.

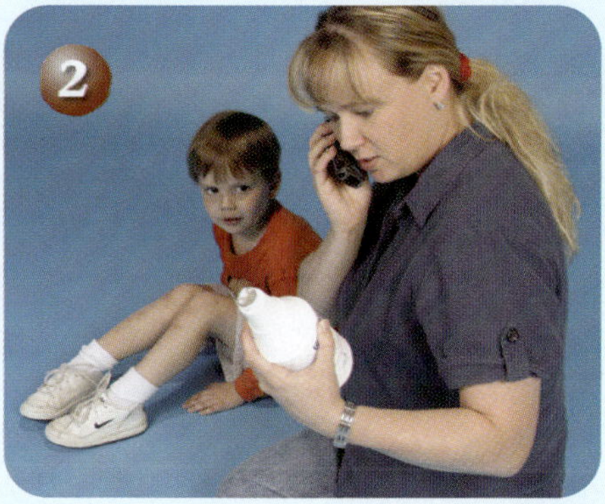

First Aid Care for Swallowed Poisons (cont.)

3. If the child is unresponsive, call EMS and follow the steps in Difficulty Breathing (page 24).

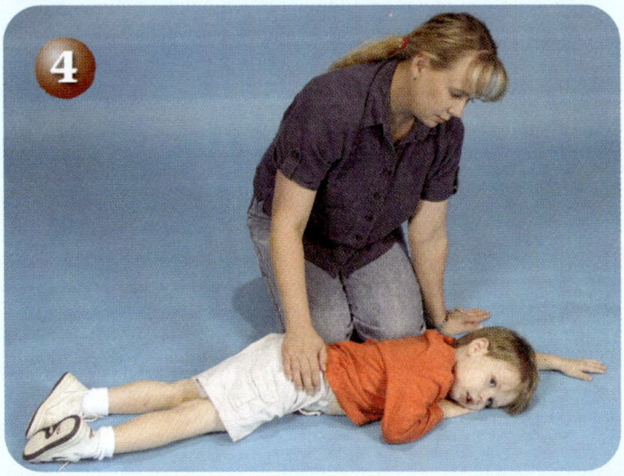

4. Place the child on his side. Lying on the left side may slow the emptying of the stomach contents. This position also keeps the airway open and allows vomit to drain from the mouth.

What You Should Do

First Aid Care for Exposure to Poisonous Plants

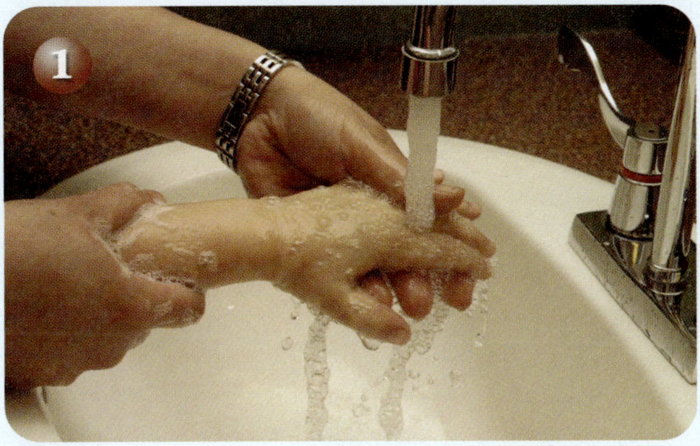

1. If a child's skin is exposed to one of these plants, immediately wash the area with soap and flush with running water to rinse off the plant oil. If a child's eye or mouth is involved, flush with water.

2. Call the poison center (800/222-1222) for further instructions.

What You Should Do

First Aid Care for Exposure to Inhaled Poisons

1. Remove the child from a toxic area and call EMS.

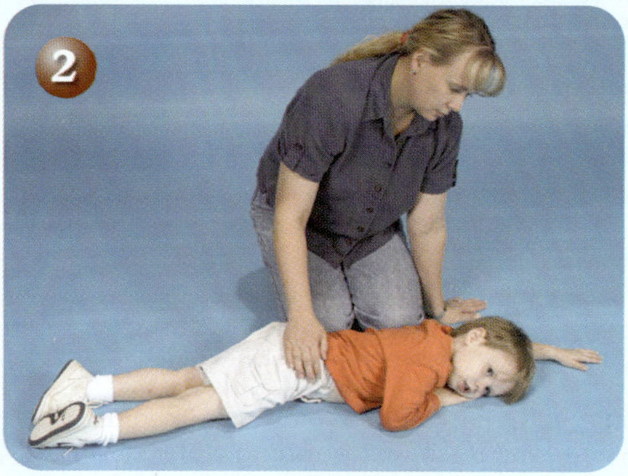

2. If the child is responsive, call the poison center (800/222-1222).

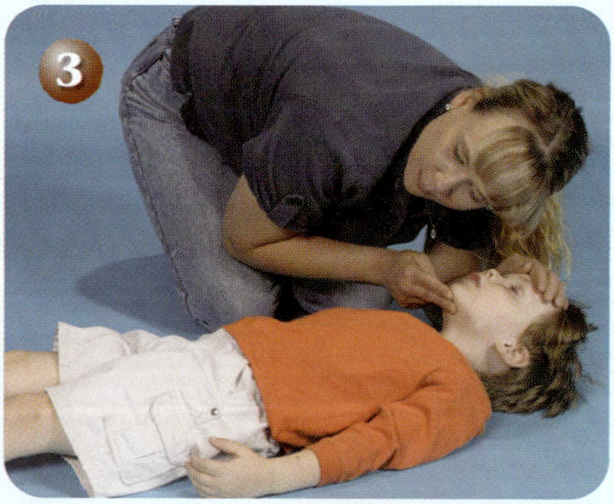

3. If the child is unresponsive follow the steps in Difficulty Breathing (page 24).

Algorithm

First Aid Care for a Swallowed Poison

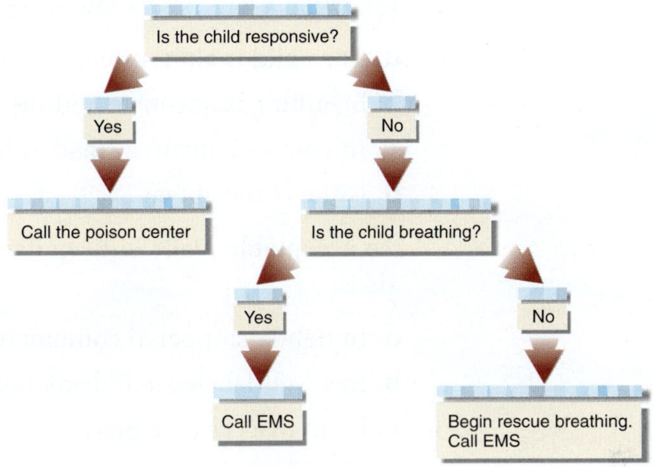

First Aid Care for an Inhaled Poison

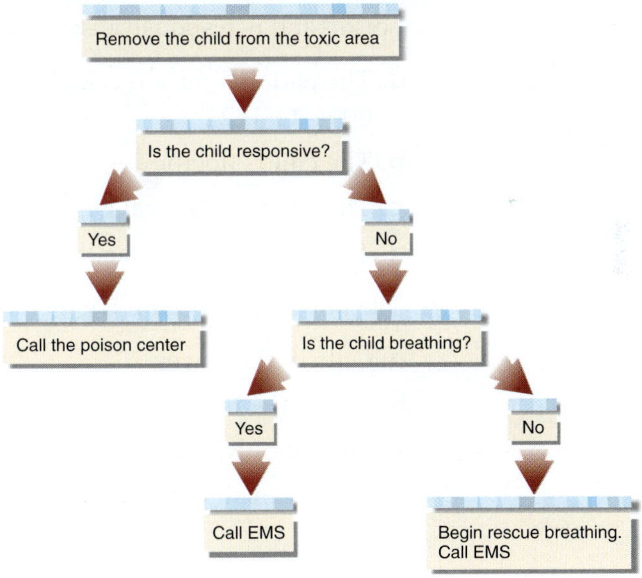

Check Your Knowledge

1. It is unnecessary to call the poison center (800/222-1222) following a child's swallowing of poisonous material if:
   a. The child is alert, oriented, and crying.
   b. Breathing is adequate and the child has good color.
   c. In your judgment, a small, safe amount was swallowed.
   d. None of the above.
2. An acceptable place to keep dangerous cleaning materials is:
   a. In tightly stoppered containers beneath the sink.
   b. In a well-labeled soft drink bottle with a tight stopper.
   c. In an inaccessible place (high, out of reach), and locked up.
   d. In a closet with the door tightly shut.
3. The first telephone call to make if a child has swallowed poison and is responsive is:
   a. The national poison center referral number, 800/222-1222.
   b. The child's doctor.
   c. The parent or a legal guardian.
   d. The director of the facility.
4. The poison in a poison ivy plant is:
   a. Only in the leaves
   b. Not in the roots
   c. Present only during the winter and fall
   d. Present in all parts of the plant

Terms

Poison A substance that, when swallowed, inhaled, or absorbed through the skin (from a plant), can cause illness, damage, and sometimes death.

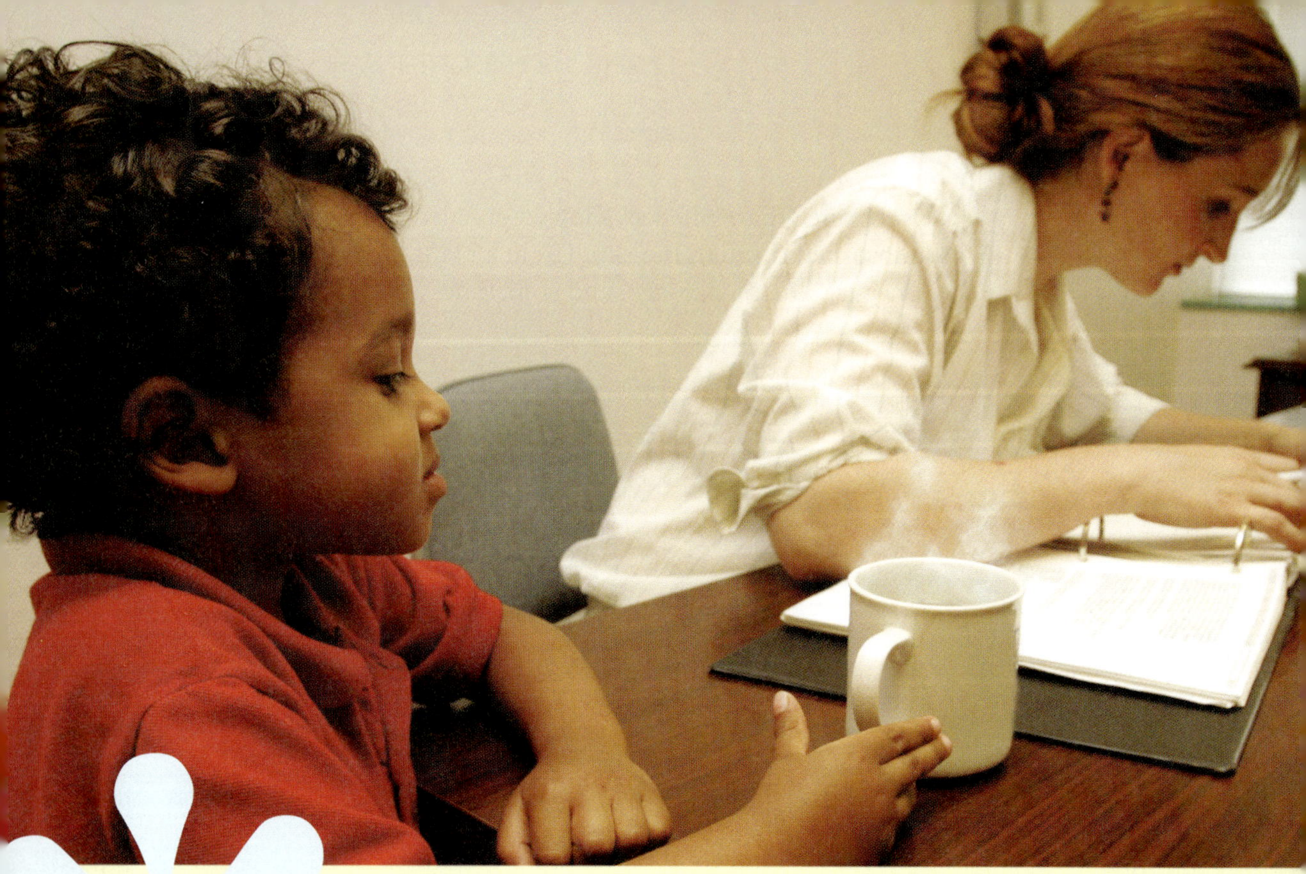

Learning Objectives

The participant will be able to:

- Identify those burns that can be addressed by first aid and those that cannot.
- Describe appropriate first aid for burns.
- Identify the symptoms of electric shock.
- Describe the appropriate first aid for electric shock.

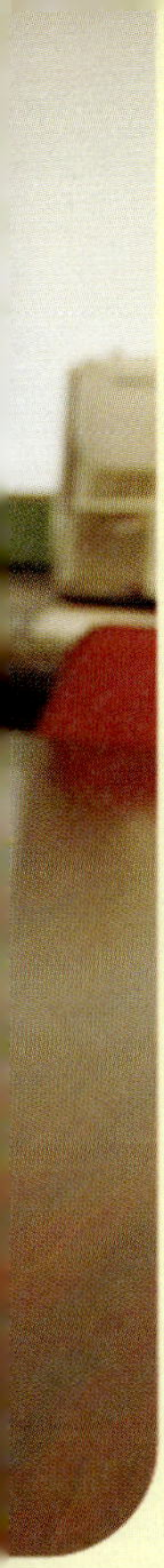

Topic 11 Burns

Burns

Introduction

A **burn** is an injury to the skin caused by heat, radiation, a chemical, or electrical damage to the body (**Figure 11-1**). Heat sources include hot water or steam, hot surfaces, and flames. Chemical burns are caused by corrosive or caustic chemicals. The most common type of radiation burn is a sunburn, which is caused by ultraviolet light. Contact with electricity causes electrical burns. Burn injuries can be very painful and may take a long time to heal. A serious burn injury can leave a child with long-term physical and emotional scars.

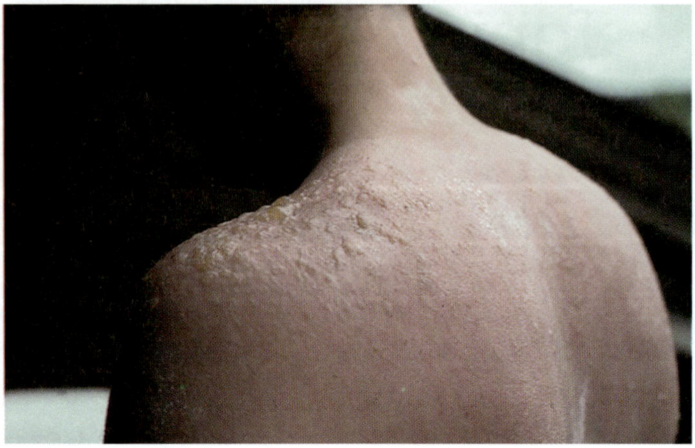

Figure 11-1

A burn is an injury to the skin.

What You Should Know

Most burns to toddlers and preschoolers are scald injuries caused by hot liquids and grease. Infants are less likely to be burned than older children due to their immobility. Burns caused by flames occur more frequently to children 5 to 12 years of age. Fires that create a lot of smoke can be damaging because the chemicals in the smoke can cause severe injury to the lining of the airway and lungs.

Did You Know ?

Temperatures above 120°F can cause serious injury to the skin within seconds. Some states have regulations that limit the temperature of water accessible to children in early education and child care facilities. You should know your state's regulations and how the issue is handled in your facility.

Corrosive or caustic chemicals cause burns by destroying the skin that comes into direct contact with the chemical. The longer the chemical is in contact with the body, the more damage it does. Some examples of corrosive or caustic chemicals are lye, drain cleaner, and battery acids. The chemical labels will tell you whether they can cause burns. These hazardous chemicals should be stored and used carefully and should be inaccessible to children.

Children are very curious and can come upon electrical dangers, such as electrical sockets and wires from appliances, while exploring (**Figure 11-2**). Toddlers may attempt to place an object, such as a fork, in an electrical socket. Infants may chew on wires. Usually children are knocked away by the strong muscle contractions that occur after contact with electricity. However, these muscle contractions can also make the child hold on to the object instead of being knocked away, thus causing more damage.

Depending on the amount of electricity, injuries can range from a minimal reddening of the skin to severe damage to the body. An electrical burn may cause substantial deep tissue injury while showing little damage on the surface of the skin. Usually, electrical shock from a household current is not life-threatening. Nevertheless, electrical shock can cause the heart to stop. If the child who is injured by electricity is still in contact with the source of the electrical current, the electricity can flow to and injure any person who touches the child.

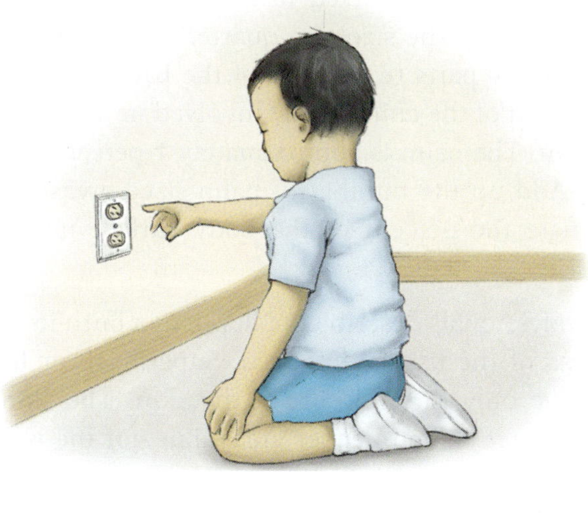

Figure 11-2

Electrical outlets should have protective devices to prevent injury.

Did You Know?

People who have a history of one or more blistering sunburns during childhood or adolescence are two times more likely to develop skin cancer. Chronic exposure to sunlight (ultraviolet light, UV) is the cause of most cases of skin cancer. More than half of a person's lifetime UV exposure occurs during childhood and adolescence. Protection from UV exposure reduces the risk for skin cancer. When children play outside, they should always wear sun-protective clothing, seek shade, and use sunscreen or sunblock. Sunscreen contains a chemical that bonds to the skin to prevent injury from UV light. Sunblock is a barrier cream that prevents the UV light from reaching the skin. Unlike burns from direct contact with hot surfaces, the irritation of the skin from sunburn takes time to develop.

The severity of a burn is determined by three major factors: size, location, and depth. The size, location, and depth of a burn determine whether a medical professional should be involved in care. Larger and deeper burns are more serious injuries. Burns of the face, hands, feet, or genitals are more serious than burns in other locations of the body. Unfortunately, children commonly burn their face, hands, feet, or genitals when they reach up to stovetops, touch hot appliances, or spill hot liquids in their laps. A burn that may be considered a minor injury to an adult could be a serious injury for a young child.

You can describe the area involved in a burn by comparison with a familiar object (e.g., "the size of a quarter") or the proportion of the involved body parts (e.g., "half of the back"). You can also estimate the percent of the child's body involved in the burn by using the child's palm. The palm is approximately 1 percent of the total body surface. Add up the number of palm-sized areas of injured skin to estimate the percent of the body surface involved (**Figure 11-3**).

Often, health professionals describe the depth of a burn in relation to the thickness of the tissues involved. Superficial, or **first-degree burns**, involve only the top part of the skin. The skin is pink, but does not blister. When deeper areas, but not the whole

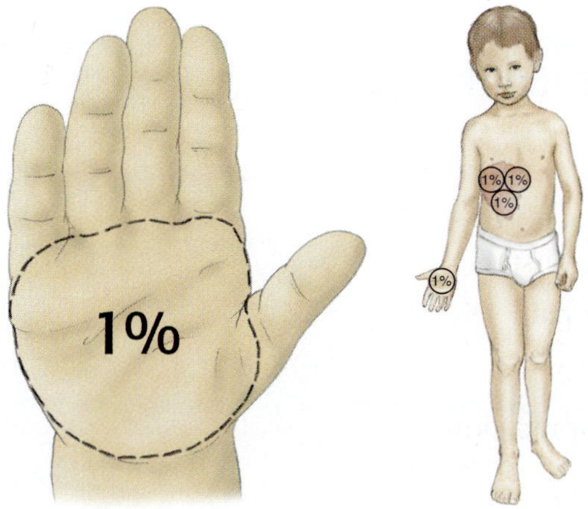

Figure 11-3

The palm is approximately 1 percent of the body surface.

thickness of the skin is burned, the injury is called a partial-thickness, or **second-degree burn**. A second-degree burn is the type that blisters. A burn that involves the full-thickness of skin may involve deeper tissues under the skin as well. This is the most serious type of burn, called a **third-degree burn**. A third-degree burn can damage the full depth of skin, muscle, and nerves (**Figure 11-4**).

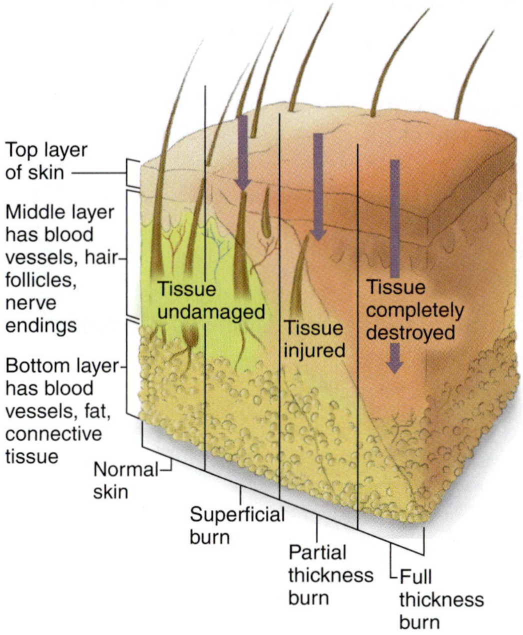

Figure 11-4

Depth of burn injury.

What You Should Look For

First-degree Burn:

- Pink or red skin
- Mild swelling, no blisters
- Mild to moderate pain

Second-degree Burn:

- Dark red or bright red skin
- Blisters
- Swelling
- Moderate to severe pain

Third-degree Burn:

- Red, raw, ash white, black, leathery, or charred skin
- Swelling
- Pain can be severe in the area surrounding a third-degree burn, although there is little or no pain in the tissues that have a third-degree burn. In the tissues involved in a third-degree burn, these nerves have been destroyed. The surrounding tissues that have only first- and second-degree burns have nerves that send pain sensations to the brain.

Chemical Burn:

- A change of color in the skin
- Pain

Electrical Burn:

- A source of electricity
- Red or white appearance to the skin that was in contact with the electricity

What You Should Do

The Eight Steps in Pediatric First Aid:

1 Survey the Scene

Take a brief moment to perform a scene survey to ensure that the scene is safe, to find out who is involved, and to determine what happened.

2 Hands-off ABCs

As you approach the child, perform the hands-off ABCs (Appearance, Breathing, and Circulation) to determine if EMS should be called. It should take 15 to 30 seconds or less.

3 Supervise

Immediately ensure that any other children near the scene are properly supervised.

4 Hands-on ABCDEs

Perform the hands-on ABCDEs (Appearance, Breathing, Circulation, Disability, and Everything else) to determine if EMS should be called and what first aid care is needed.

5 First Aid Care

Provide first aid care appropriate to the injury or illness.

6 Notify

As soon as possible, notify the child's parent(s) or legal guardian(s).

7 Debrief

As soon as possible, talk with the child who received first aid about any concerns he or she may have, and talk with other children who witnessed the injury and first aid procedures.

8 Document

Complete an incident report form.

First Aid Tip

You should provide first aid care for all burns, but the child needs to see a medical professional as soon as possible for:

- Burns of the face, hands, or genitals.
- Burns that cover more than 1 percent of the body surface.
- All electrical injuries.

What You Should Do

First Aid Care for Burns from Heat Sources, Including Sunburn

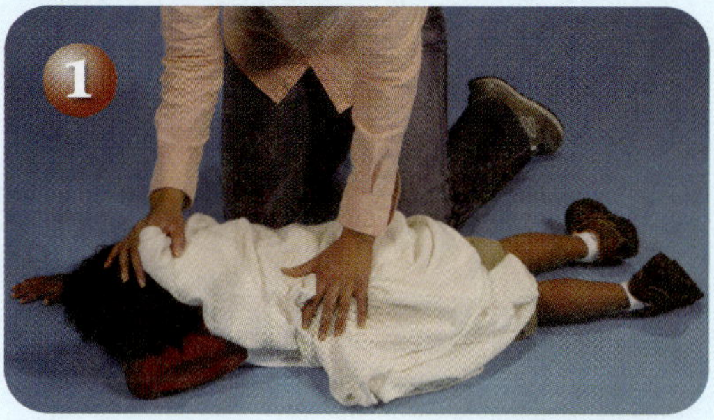

1 Stop the heat injury by removing child from contact with the source of heat, sunshine, or whatever is causing the burn. If flames are present, smother them by using a blanket or rolling the child on the floor or ground. Prevent the child from running because this fans the flames. Call EMS if the burn includes injured areas that are raw, ash white, black, leathery, or charred (third-degree burns), if the burn involves the face, hands, feet, or genitals, or if the burn is more than 1% of the body surface.

2 Unless a very large part of the body is involved, use cool water right away to take the heat out of the body tissues and reduce the pain in the injured area. You should cool a first-, second-, or third-degree burn even if it involves a large area. For areas that are larger than the palm of the child's hand (larger than 1 percent), limit cooling to an area that is no bigger than 3 times the size of the child's palm for 1 to 2 minutes at a time, and then move to another area. This approach will avoid chilling the whole body. You should continue to cool a burn, even one that is a third-degree burn, until the pain stops or the child gets medical care.

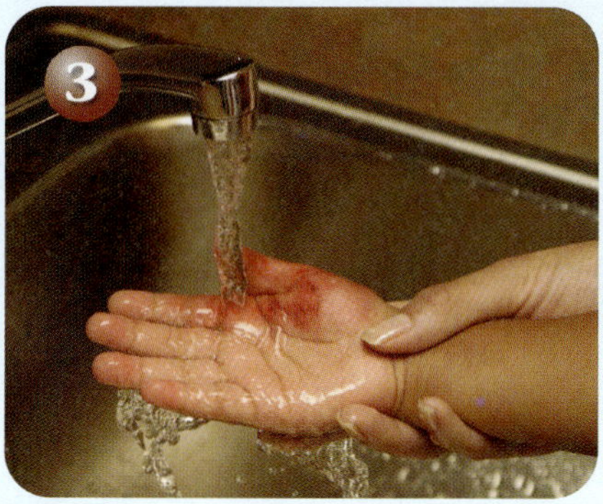

3 To cool a burn, you can place the burned area in a container of cool water or let a gentle (not forceful) flow of cool tap water run over the burned area. Sometimes children will cooperate with this first aid care if they are allowed to play in the cool water with a few toys. If you cannot put the burned area into cool water, (e.g., a burn on the face) cover it with a cold, wet towel, rewetting or replacing the towel every 1 to 2 minutes to keep the towel cool. Another approach is to put a cold pack on top of a wet towel covering the injured area.

First Aid Care for Burns from Heat Sources, Including Sunburn (cont.)

4. Prevent chilling of the child from cooling a burn by removing any wet clothing that is not helping to cool the burned area. Do not remove clothing that is stuck to the skin. If wet clothing is stuck to skin, cut around the stuck area to remove the wet clothing that is not stuck to the skin. Leave the clothing that is stuck to the skin alone. Then cover unburned areas with a sheet or blankets as needed to keep the child comfortably warm while keeping the burned area cool.

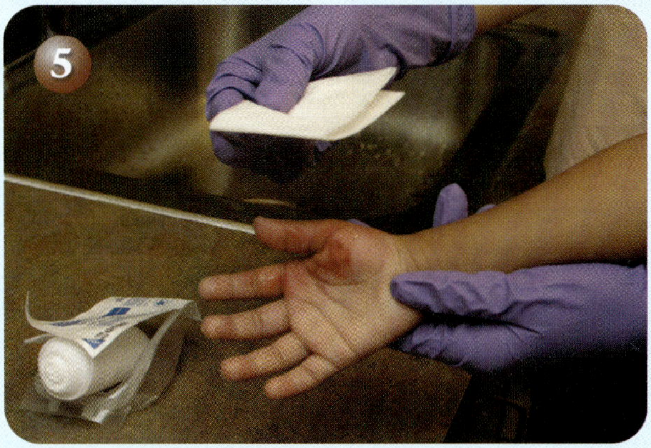

5. Apply a loosely fitted dressing over the burned area, after cooling the burn until the pain stops.

What You Should Do

First Aid Care for Chemical Burns

1. Stop the injury by removing the child from contact with the chemical.

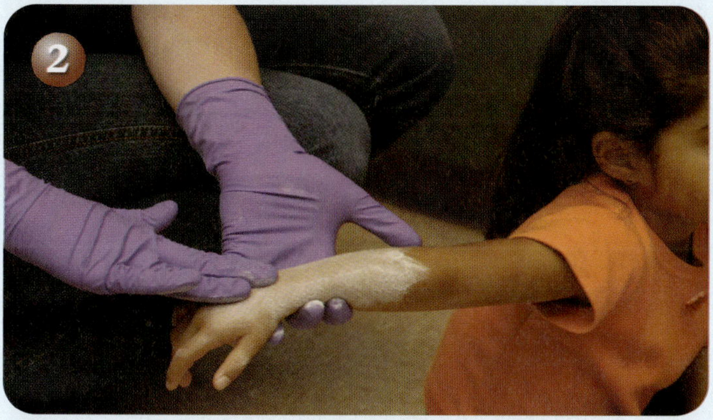

2. Brush off any dry chemical that remains on the skin. Remove constricting items such as jewelry.

3. Call EMS.

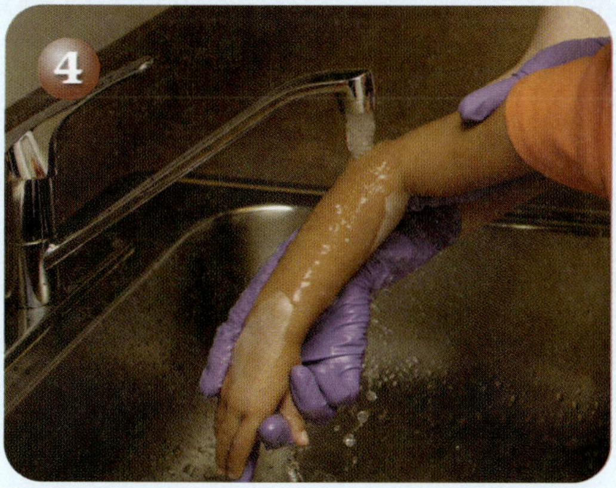

4. Rinse the area of the body that was in contact with the chemical with a continuous gentle flow of fresh water over the entire affected area for 15 to 20 minutes.

What You Should Do

First Aid Care for Electrical Burns

1. Be sure that the child is no longer connected to the source of the electricity. Turn off the power source before approaching the child. If you are unable turn off the power source, push/pull the victim away from the source of electricity with thick dry cloth or wood stick (broom handle or chair) or a dry towel looped around the child's feet.

2. Call EMS.

First Aid Tip

- Always cover ice before putting it on a burn. Direct application of ice to body tissues can damage fragile tissues that remain.
- Do not apply burn ointments, petroleum jelly, margarine, toothpaste or anything other than fresh cool water as first aid care for a burn. A medical professional should prescribe any medications that are used on a burn.
- Keep blisters from breaking if you can. An unbroken blister is a sterile dressing over the injured tissue that helps to prevent infection. When the blister breaks, germs can get into the damaged tissues and grow. After the cooling step is completed, place a loose protective dressing over the blisters to try to keep them from breaking.

Algorithm

First Aid Care for Burns

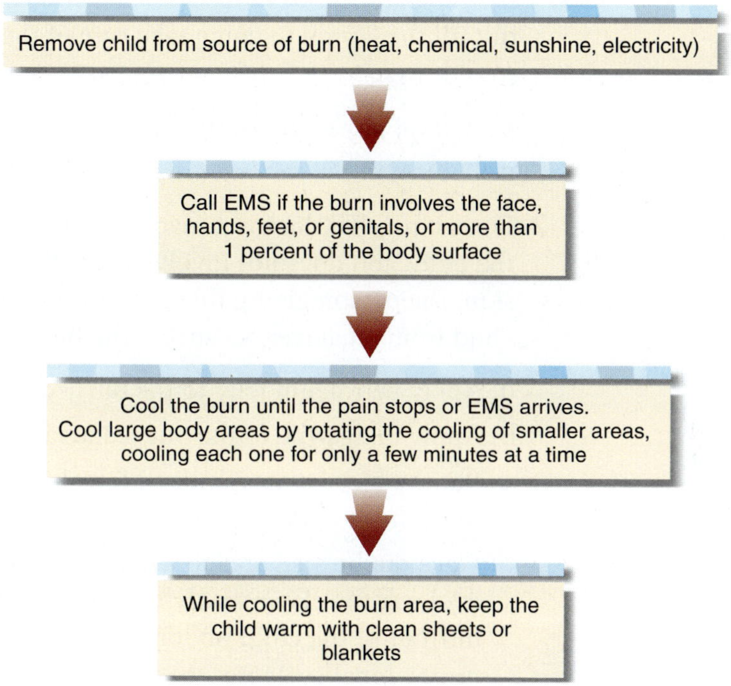

Check Your Knowledge

1. If a burn involves the face, hands, feet, genitals, or a large area of the body, the person giving first aid should:

a. Call the family to come take care of the child.

b. Call EMS.

c. Pull off any clothing that is stuck to the wound.

d. Put ice on the injured area.

2. For a burn that does not involve more than 1 percent of the body, and does not involve the full thickness of the skin, the person giving first aid care should remove the child from whatever is causing the burn and then:

a. Apply petroleum jelly to the burned area.

b. Apply margarine to the burned area.

c. Put the burned area under a forceful stream of cool water from the faucet.

d. Place the burned area in a container of cool water or use cool wet towels or gently running water to cool the burn until the child no longer has pain or a medical professional evaluates the child's burn.

3. For a child who is outside and appears to have sunburn, you should first:

a. Remove the child from exposure to sunlight.

b. Comfort the child.

c. Put a hat on the child.

d. Put ice on the sunburn.

4. When blisters form in the area of the burn the person providing first aid should:

a. Wipe off a sewing needle with alcohol and puncture the blister so the fluid drains out.

b. Press on the blister to see if the fluid will drain from it.

c. Wash the blister with soap and water and then cover it with petroleum jelly.

d. Cover the blister with a loose, protective dressing to try to keep the blister intact.

Terms

Burn	An injury to the skin that results from heat, radiation, a chemical, or electrical damage to the body.
First-degree burns	Burns that involve only the top part of the skin.
Second-degree burns	Burns that blister and involve a deeper thickness of the skin.
Third-degree burns	Burns that involve the entire thickness of the skin and deeper tissue.

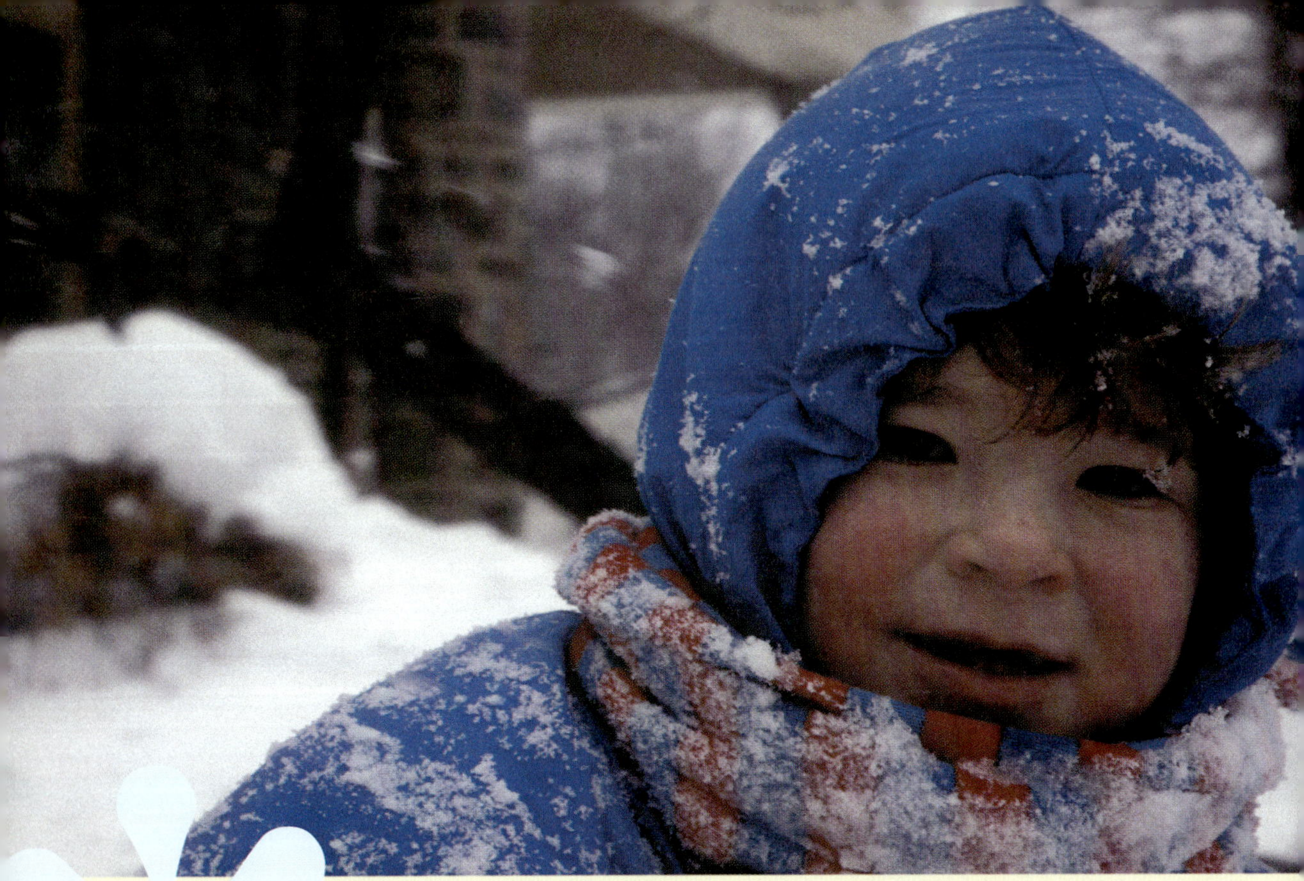

Learning Objectives

The participant will be able to:

- Describe a child who is having a cold-related injury (frostbite, hypothermia).
- Describe appropriate first aid for a child who is having a cold-related injury.
- Recognize heat-related injuries (heat stroke, heat exhaustion, heat cramps, dehydration).
- Identify appropriate first aid for a child who is having a heat-related injury.

Topic

12 Heat- and Cold-Related Injuries

Heat- and Cold-Related Injuries

Introduction

Infants and small children are more vulnerable to injury from the extremes of heat and cold than adults. Children get chilled and overheated more quickly than adults. Children are also less aware of the dangers from the heat and cold.

Injury from extremes of heat and cold is not only related to temperature but also to factors such as humidity, wind, clothing, and length of exposure. Two terms that help describe the risk of injury from heat and cold are **wind chill** and **heat index.** Wind chill is the difference between the actual temperature and how cold it feels. The wind carries heat away from the body, cooling it more rapidly than would otherwise occur. The heat index is how hot it feels because of humidity and temperature. At higher levels of humidity, it is harder for perspiration to evaporate. Without cooling of the body by evaporation of sweat, it is easier for the body to become overheated.

Heat-Related Illness

What You Should Know

The body produces heat constantly. The body produces more heat during exercise and sometimes during illness. When body temperatures exceed the normal body temperature (98.6°F), the body has a fever. Normally, in an environment without excessive heat, body temperatures from illness will not exceed 106°F. Temperatures above 106°F can cause permanent harm to the body.

When it is hot, cooling is largely accomplished by the evaporation of sweat. If the air is already humid, sweat does not evaporate quickly, so cooling by sweating becomes less efficient. Some children do not sweat enough to cool themselves as well as other children. Wearing fabrics that trap sweat can restrict cooling.

Usually, the first signs of excess body heat are nausea, headache, and disorientation. If the body temperature does not go down, brain damage and death can occur. The most severe form of heat illness is **heatstroke.** When heatstroke occurs, the body's heat-regulating ability becomes overwhelmed and ceases to function properly, resulting in an inability to sweat and a dangerously high rise in body temperature.

Heatstroke can develop suddenly. An infant or child with heatstroke will have a body temperature of 106°F or higher. Once the ability of the sweat glands to produce sweat is exhausted, the skin may be dry and hot. Often, the skin is flushed. Rapid breathing is present. Usually, confusion or loss of consciousness occurs. Heatstroke is far more common among the elderly and in athletes, but can occur in an active child or in an infant who is overly clothed and insufficiently cooled off.

Heat exhaustion is the result of prolonged exposure to a hot environment, often while actively playing and sweating. Heat exhaustion is largely the result of dehydration from failing to drink a sufficient amount of water to replace fluid that is lost through sweating (**Figure 12-1**). **Heat cramps** are painful muscle spasms, often in the legs. Heat cramps are the result of dehydration in the body caused by insufficient replacement of water lost by sweating.

A child suffering from heat exhaustion will be thirsty and sweating heavily. Pay attention to how often children are urinating during hot conditions and what color the urine is. If the urine is dark and the child is not urinating at least once every 4 hours, you can prevent dehydration by encouraging the child to drink more often, even if the child only drinks a small amount at a time. A child who has heat exhaustion may feel weak, nauseated, and very tired. There is little or no elevation of the body temperature at this stage of heat illness. The child's tongue and mouth are likely to look dry. Heat cramps may accompany heat exhaustion. A child may complain of muscle cramps, usually in the legs and abdominal muscles.

Did You Know?

In the summer of 2003, a severe heat wave occurred in France and other parts of Europe. Over 10,000 people died in France of heatstroke. All ages were involved, but most of the victims were elderly.

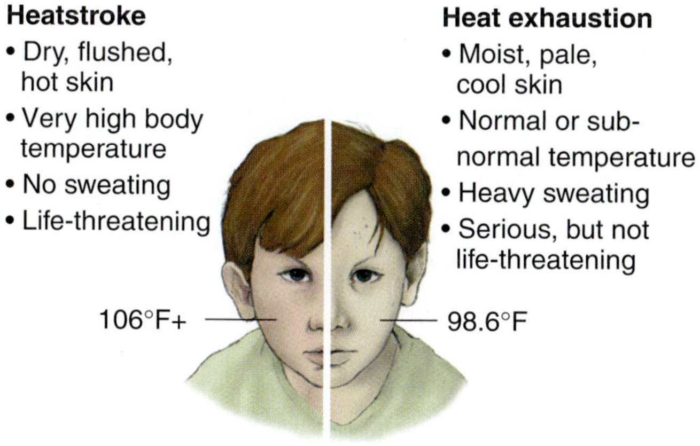

Figure 12-1

Comparison between heat stroke and heat exhaustion.

What You Should Look For

- Heavy sweating for more than a short time, or no sweating when the environment is hot
- Looks and acts ill or more tired than expected; an older child complains of nausea or headache
- Not urinating at least once every 4 hours and not drinking very often when the environment is hot
- Skin is flushed, especially the face
- Disoriented, confused
- Breathing rapidly
- Body temperature is elevated

What You Should Do

The Eight Steps in Pediatric First Aid:

1 Survey the Scene

Take a brief moment to perform a scene survey to ensure that the scene is safe, to find out who is involved, and to determine what happened.

2 Hands-off ABCs

As you approach the child, perform the hands-off ABCs (Appearance, Breathing, and Circulation) to determine if EMS should be called. It should take 15 to 30 seconds or less.

3 Supervise

Immediately ensure that any other children near the scene are properly supervised.

4 Hands-on ABCDEs

Perform the hands-on ABCDEs (Appearance, Breathing, Circulation, Disability, and Everything else) to determine if EMS should be called and what first aid care is needed.

5 First Aid Care

Provide first aid care appropriate to the injury or illness.

6 Notify

As soon as possible, notify the child's parent(s) or legal guardian(s).

7 Debrief

As soon as possible, talk with the child who received first aid about any concerns he or she may have, and talk with other children who witnessed the injury and first aid procedures.

8 Document

Complete an incident report form.

What You Should Do

First Aid Care for Heatstroke

1. Cool the child immediately and call EMS.

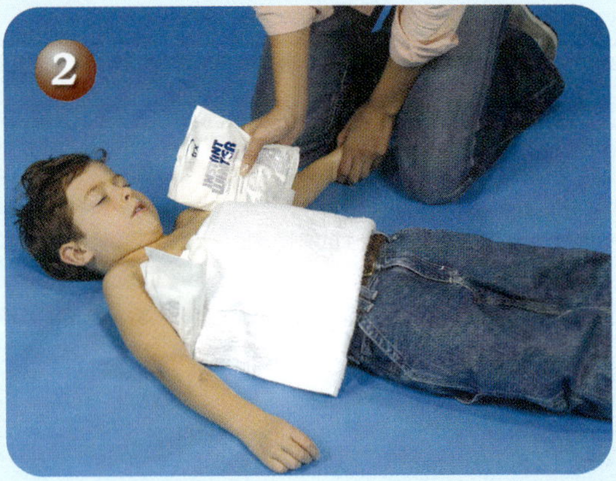

2. Cooling is best accomplished by pouring lots of cool water over the child. If the child tolerates it, put ice packs or ice wrapped in a wet cloth in the armpits and groin of the child. This will cool the blood that goes through the big blood vessels close to the skin in those areas.

What You Should Do

First Aid Care for Heat Exhaustion and Heat Cramps

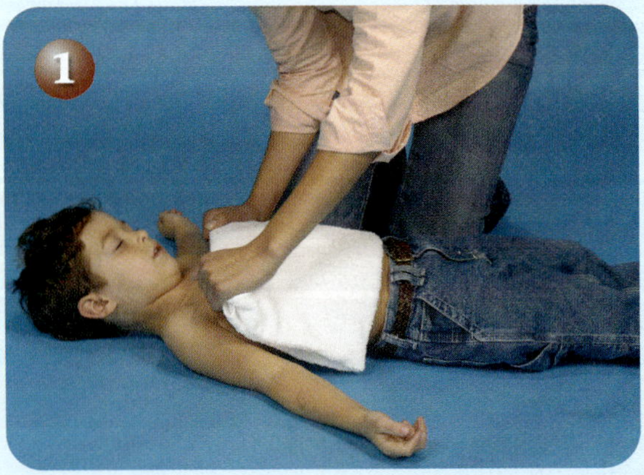

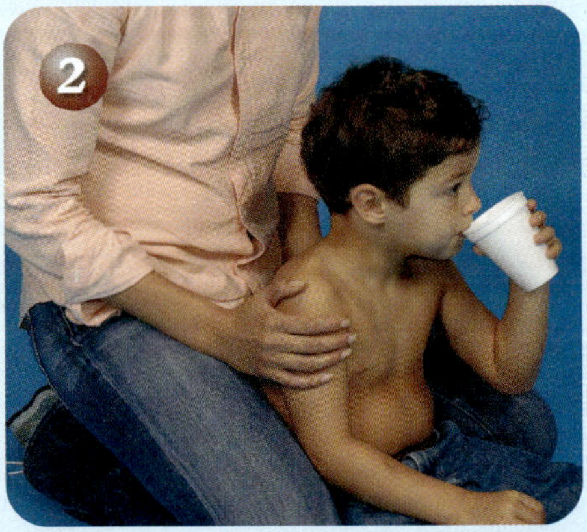

1. Move the child into a cool place. If a cool place is not available, cool the child's body by pouring cool water over the skin or use wet cool cloths. Continue to rinse and reapply cool cloths after they become warmed by contact with the body.

2. Encourage the child to drink of lots of water. The "sports drinks" are not better than water, and water is more readily available.

Cold-Related Injuries

What You Should Know

Hypothermia is a dangerous condition in which, through severe exposure to cold, the core body temperature (the temperature deep within the body) drops below 95°F. Body processes slow at these low temperatures and tissue damage can occur. The cause of hypothermia is prolonged exposure to the cold. Falling into cold water is a common cause, as is being outside too long without proper clothing during cold weather. Body temperatures drop when the body is unable to produce enough heat to compensate for heat loss. The outside temperature does not have to be below freezing for hypothermia to occur.

Frostbite is tissue damage caused by extreme cold (**Figure 12-2**). Ears, face, hands, and feet are especially susceptible because tissues in these areas are thin, exposed, or are far from the body core. **Frostnip** is the most common local cold injury. There is minimal tissue damage and no actual freezing of the tissue.

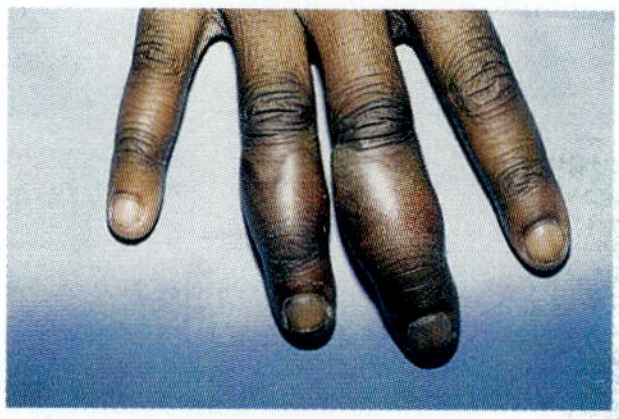

Figure 12-2

Frostbite.

What You Should Look For

- Body temperature is lower than normal
- Child is sluggish and may be unconscious
- Injured skin with frostnip or frostbite appears cold, pale, and feels numb to the touch
- Injured skin may blister
- When body part is warmed, tissues that have been injured may have more blood in them than usual, may turn pink, or if the damage is severe, may remain pale
- Mild to moderately damaged tissues hurt, tingle, and feel like they are burning

What You Should Do

First Aid Care for Hypothermia

1. Bring the child into a warm place and call EMS. Until you can get to a warm room, bring the child close to someone else's warm body.

2. Strip off the cold wet clothes and replace them with warm dry ones.

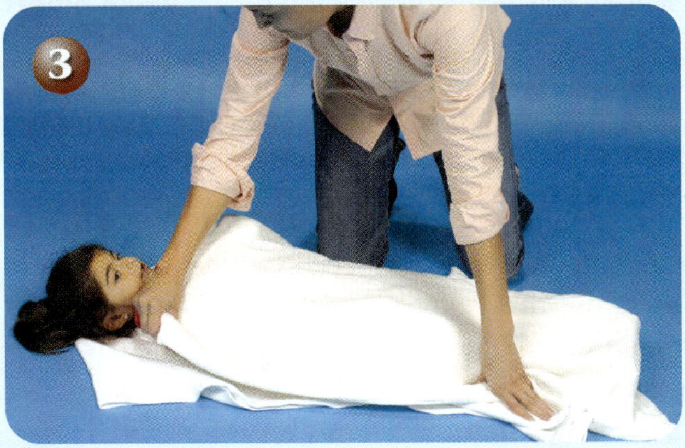

3. Wrap the child in a blanket.

What You Should Do

First Aid Care for Frostbite and Frostnip

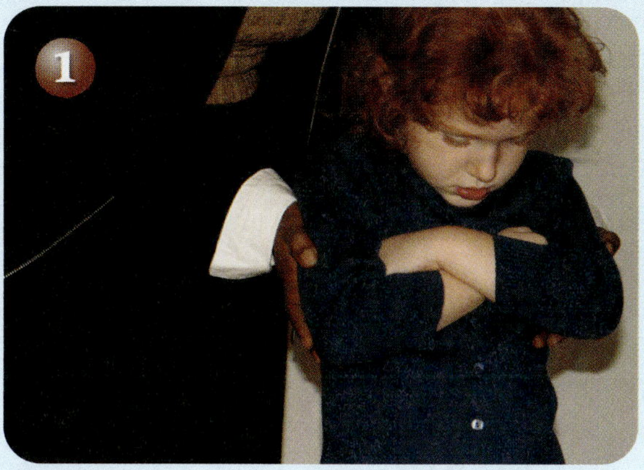

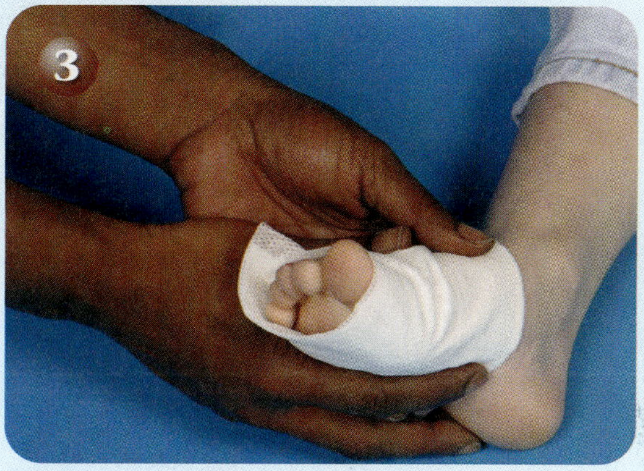

1. Take the child to a warm room and call EMS. Until you can get to a warm room, place cold body parts close to warm body areas. For example, tuck cold hands into the armpits.

2. Remove any wet clothes including shoes and socks, and cover the areas with clean, warm, and dry coverings.

3. Do not break any blisters that may be present, but cover those that have broken with gauze.

4. Allow the cold-injured part to return to normal body temperature slowly.

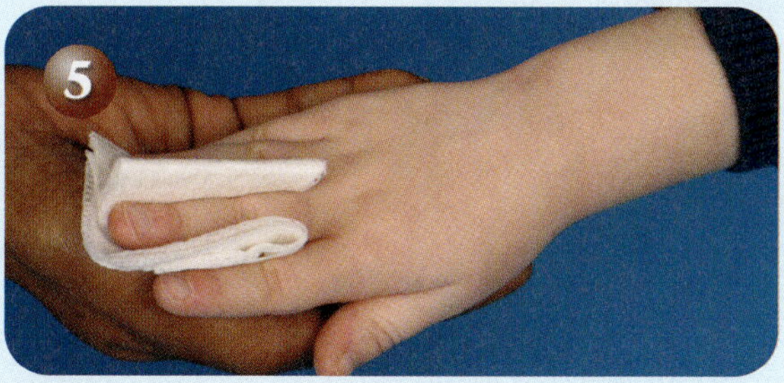

5. If toes or fingers are cold damaged, put dry gauze between the toes or fingers to keep them from rubbing each other.

6. Inform the child's parent(s) or legal guardian(s) that the child may need medical attention.

Algorithm

First Aid Care for Heat-Related Illness

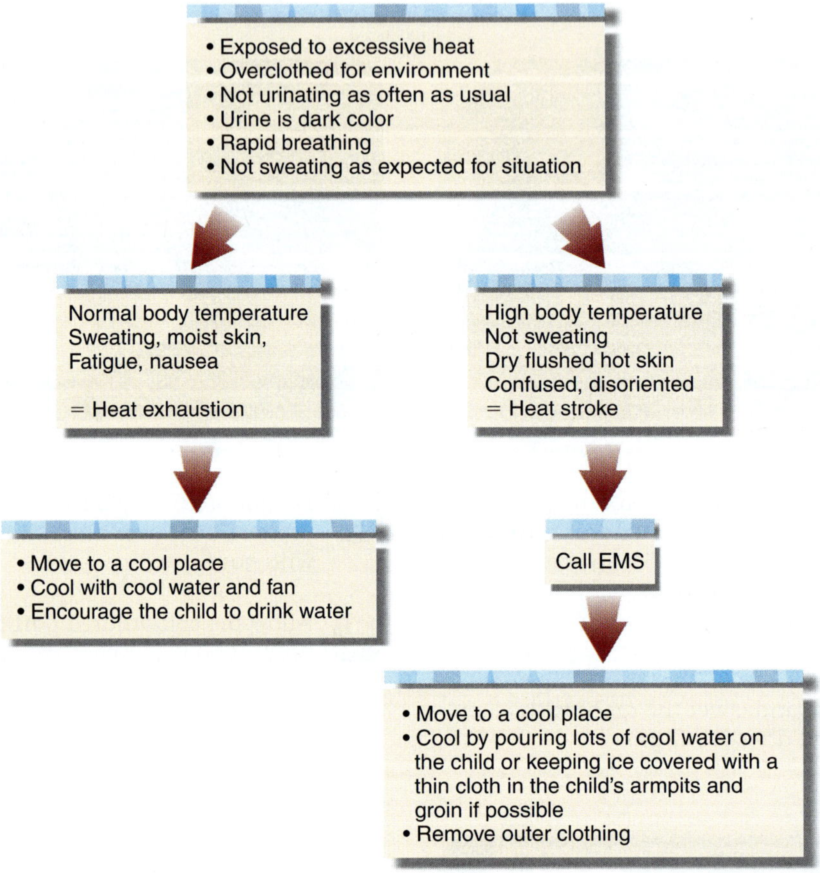

First Aid Care for Hypothermia

Chilled, cold
Sluggish behavior

↓

Call EMS

↓

- Move child to warm area
- Strip cold and wet clothing, including shoes and socks
- Replace with warm dry clothing and/or blanket

First Aid Care for Frostbite

Cold body part, skin blisters, swollen, hard skin

↓

- Remove cold and wet clothing, including shoes and socks
- Cover with warm clothing and blanket
- Contact the parent(s) or legal guardian(s) and inform them that their child may need medical attention

Check Your Knowledge

1. In the event of frostbite you should:

   a. Rub the affected part, with snow if possible, to restore circulation.

   b. Take the child to a warm room, remove any wet clothing, and cover with clean, warm, dry coverings.

   c. Warm the affected part with hot water.

   d. Get the child something warm to drink.

2. A heavily dressed, very active child appears confused one summer day. Her skin is hot and dry. Her temperature is 106°F. What should you do?

   a. Insist that she drink two large glasses of a sports drink.

   b. Immediately bring the child inside, call EMS, and cool by continuously pouring cold water on her.

   c. Get someone to find a hose or small basin to cool her hands and feet.

   d. Pour a little cool water for her to drink slowly.

3. Heat exhaustion:

   a. Is largely a matter of dehydration and inability of sweating to cool the body off in a hot environment.

   b. Is the result of having consumed too much water while playing out of doors.

   c. Is best treated by letting the child rest in the shade.

   d. Is the result of lying around on a hot and humid day.

4. Hypothermia:

   a. Does not cause problems in children because their bodies are small and they move around a lot.

   b. Is caused by prolonged exposure to the cold.

   c. Is unlikely to cause permanent damage, because children so quickly recover.

   d. Causes the child to develop a high fever.

Terms

Frostbite Tissue damage caused by extreme cold.

Frostnip The most common local cold injury. There is minimal tissue damage and no actual freezing of tissue.

Heat cramps Painful muscle spasms, often in the legs. The result of dehydration in the body caused by insufficient replacement of water lost by sweating.

Heat exhaustion The result of prolonged exposure to a hot environment, often while actively playing and sweating.

Heat index The difference between the actual temperature and how hot it feels because of humidity and temperature.

Heatstroke The body's heat-regulating ability becomes overwhelmed and ceases to function properly, resulting in an inability to sweat and a dangerously high rise in body temperature.

Hypothermia A dangerous condition in which, through severe exposure to cold, the core body temperature drops below 95°F.

Wind chill The difference between the actual temperature and how cold it feels.

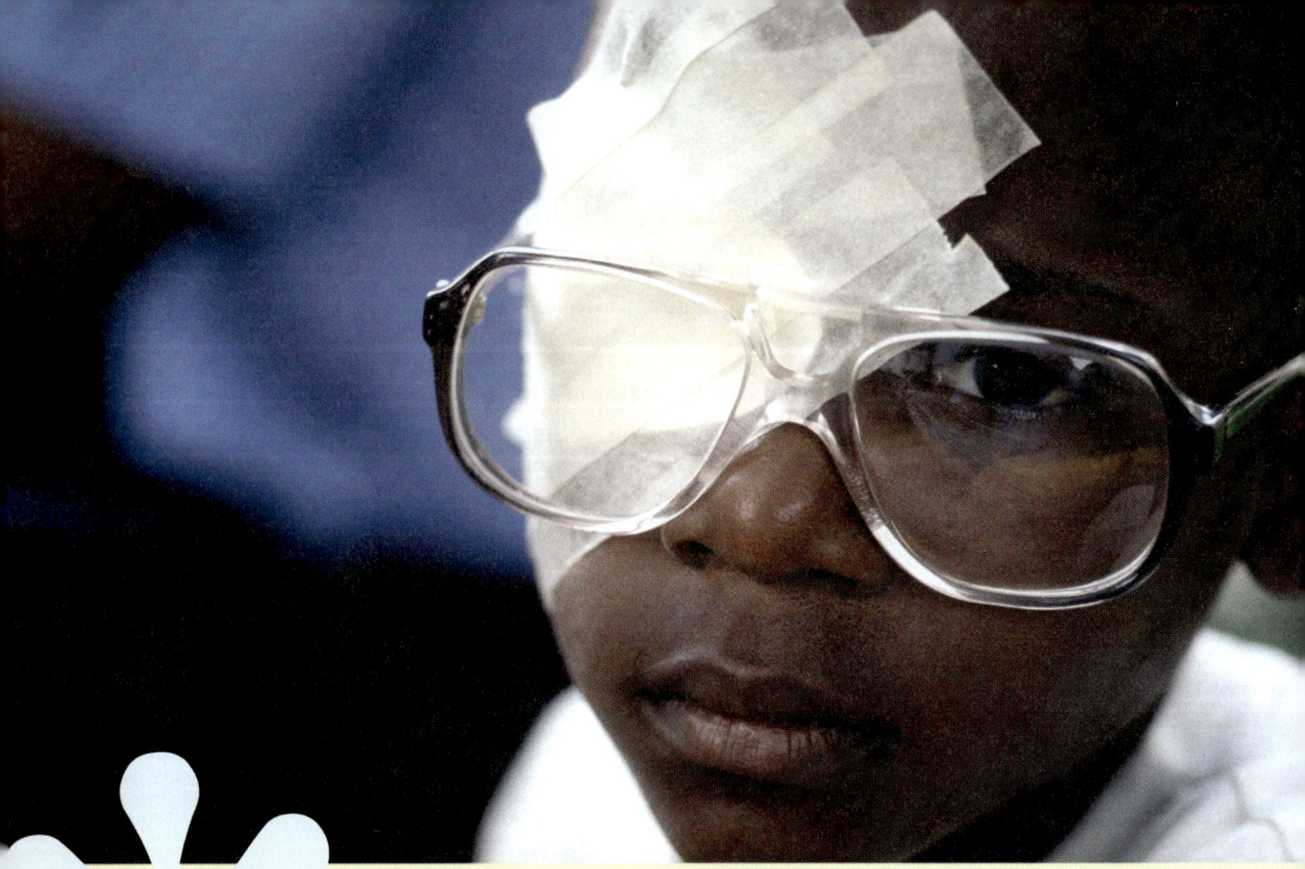

Learning Objectives

The participant will be able to:

- Recognize eye injuries in a child care setting.
- List first aid needed for eye injuries in a child care setting.

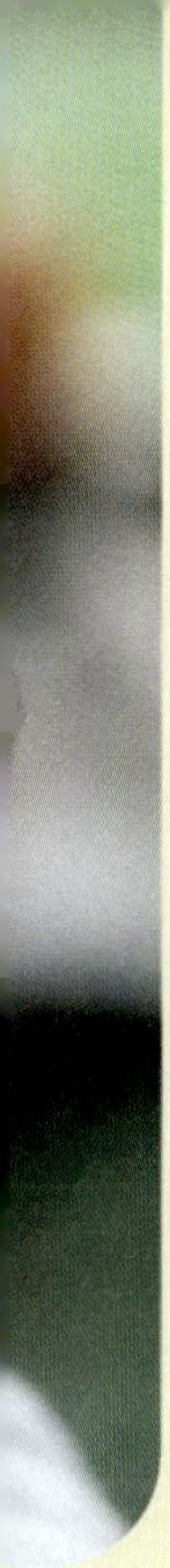

Topic 13 Eye Injuries

Eye Injuries

Introduction

An **eye injury** includes injury to the eye, eyelid, and area around the eye. Common eye injuries result from scratches, cuts, foreign bodies, burns, chemicals, and blows to the eye. The main concern when a child has suffered from an eye injury is possible damage to the child's vision. Eye injuries are the most common and preventable causes of blindness.

What You Should Know

Eye trauma refers to any injury to the eye. Eye trauma occurs often in children and is a common cause of loss of vision. According to the National Society to Prevent Blindness, approximately 1/3 of eye loss in children under 10 years of age is due to trauma to the eye. Activities that are commonly associated with eye trauma include: archery, hockey, darts, BB guns, bicycling, baseball, boxing, basketball, and sports that involve rackets. Fingernails, toys, and chemicals are also common causes of trauma. Each year, toys and home playground equipment cause more than 11,000 injuries to young eyes.

What You Should Look For

- Double vision
- Decrease in vision
- Sensitivity to light
- Redness or swelling
- Pain when moving the eye in any direction
- Blood in the eye (hemorrhage)
- Dizziness
- Numbness
- Inability to open eye after trauma

Any of the above symptoms indicate that this child should receive immediate medical attention.

What You Should Do

The Eight Steps in Pediatric First Aid:

1 Survey the Scene

Take a brief moment to perform a scene survey to ensure that the scene is safe, to find out who is involved, and to determine what happened.

2 Hands-off ABCs

As you approach the child, perform the hands-off ABCs (Appearance, Breathing, and Circulation) to determine if EMS should be called. It should take 15 to 30 seconds or less.

3 Supervise

Immediately ensure that any other children near the scene are properly supervised.

4 Hands-on ABCDEs

Perform the hands-on ABCDEs (Appearance, Breathing, Circulation, Disability, and Everything else) to determine if EMS should be called and what first aid care is needed.

5 First Aid Care

Provide first aid care appropriate to the injury or illness.

6 Notify

As soon as possible, notify the child's parent(s) or legal guardian(s).

7 Debrief

As soon as possible, talk with the child who received first aid about any concerns he or she may have, and talk with other children who witnessed the injury and first aid procedures.

8 Document

Complete an incident report form.

What You Should Do

First Aid Care for Chemical Injury to the Eye

1. Wear disposable gloves and immediately flush the chemical from the eye with lukewarm water.

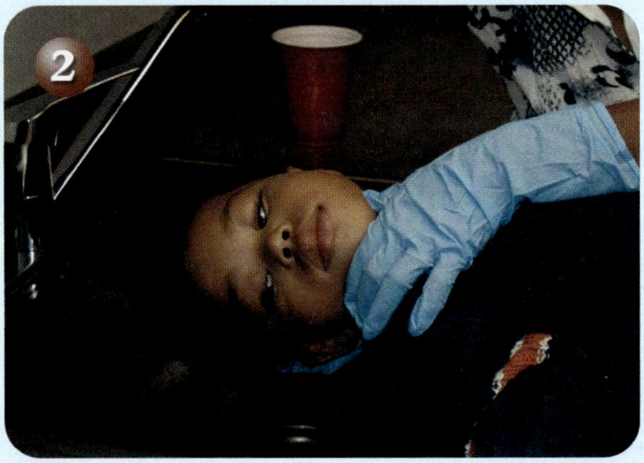

2. Position the head over a sink with the injured eye down to prevent the rinse water from contaminating the other eye.

3. Hold the injured eye open with your fingers and flush with water for 15 minutes.

4. Rinse from the inside of the eye toward the outside. You may need to securely hold the child still.

5. Have someone call the poison center (800/222-1222) while you flush the eye.

6. Inform the child's parent(s) or legal guardian(s) that the child should be seen by a health care professional.

Did You Know

Chemicals get into children's eyes most commonly from products in spray bottles, such as household cleaners and pesticides. A chemical burn to the eye requires immediate first aid treatment to prevent damage to the **cornea,** the transparent outer covering of the eyeball. Eye damage can occur swiftly—in less than 5 minutes. Certain chemical agents can cause rapid and severe damage. The eye may not appear red, but vision may be threatened.

What You Should Do

First Aid Care for Penetrating Injury to the Eye

1. Call EMS.

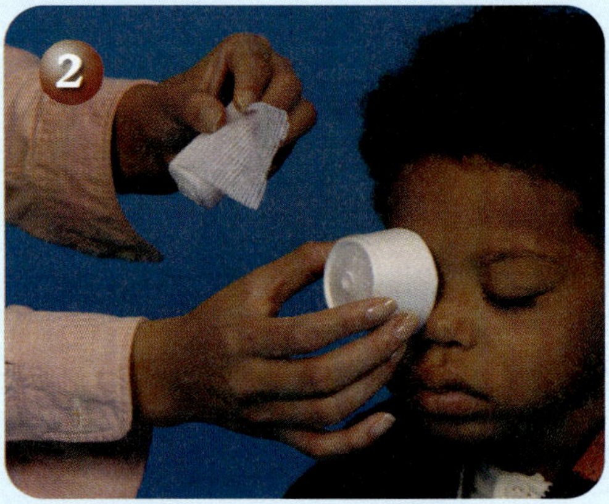

2. Penetrating eye injuries generally include lacerations, or open wounds in the eye. Attempt to cover the injured eye with an eye shield, paper cup, or even cardboard folded into a cone. If the child strongly resists covering the eye, do not insist.

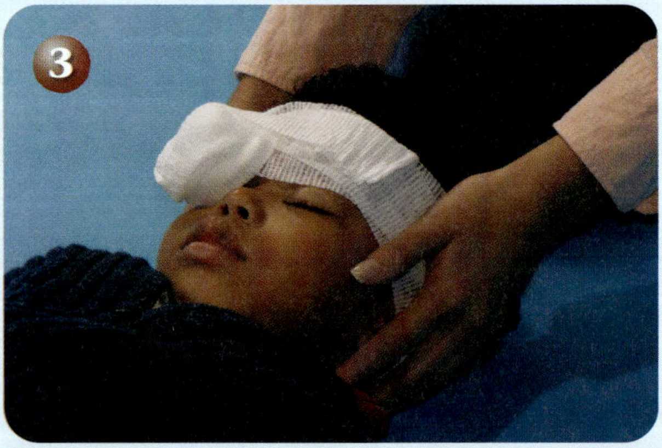

3. Keep the child as quiet as possible. The best position is for the child to lie still and be flat on his back, but do not force the child to lie in this position if he resists. Never attempt to remove a foreign object penetrating the eye, since this may cause more damage than the initial injury. Never apply pressure to the eye. Do not apply medication or preparations.

What You Should Do

First Aid Care for Foreign Object in the Eye

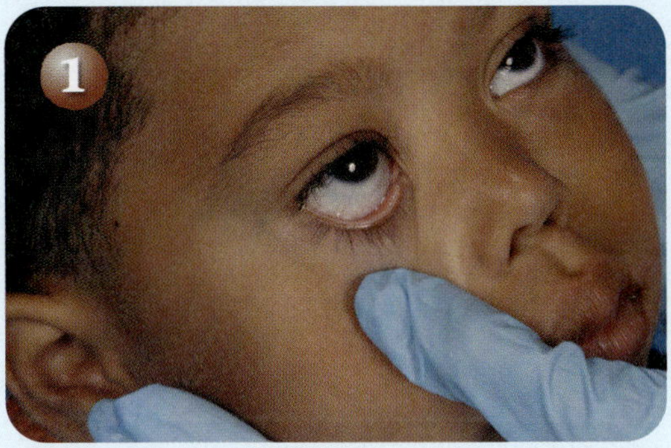

1 A foreign body can be any material (e.g., dust, sand, paint) which gets into the eye. Wear disposable gloves and pull down the child's lower eyelid to look at the inner surface while the child looks up. A speck of dirt can usually be removed with a clean wet gauze or handkerchief.

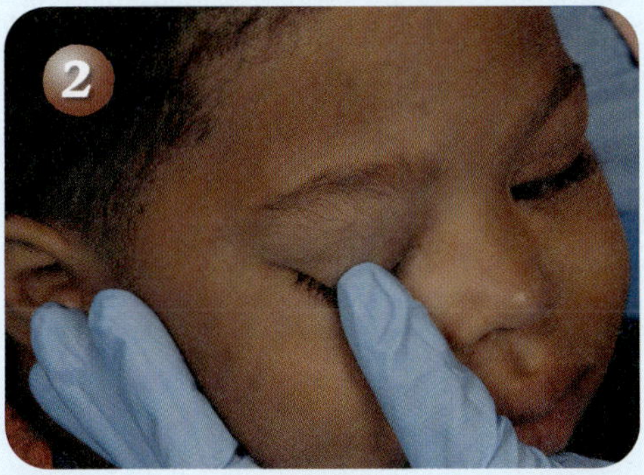

2 Gently grasp the upper lid and pull it out and down over the lower eyelid. Tears that occur when you pull the upper lid over the lower lid may help dislodge the object.

3 If the object remains, flush the eye with water. Position the head over a sink, injured eye down. Hold the eye open with your fingers and use an unbreakable cup to rinse from the inside (nose side) of the eye toward the outside (ear side) of the eye. Do not apply medication.

4 The child should be examined by a health care professional if the eye continues to tear or be red or painful. The foreign body might have scratched the cornea, and this injury can only be confirmed by a professional with a special dye and medical equipment.

Did You Know?

Eye lashes, dirt, insects, and bits of sand are foreign objects that commonly cause discomfort, redness, and tearing of the eyes. If a child has a foreign object in the eye, rubbing the eye can scratch the cornea. A scratch of the cornea is commonly called a **corneal abrasion.** A corneal abrasion is very painful, and can lead to a threatening infection. Covering an injured eye may reduce some of the pain, but it will not heal the injury. Do not force the child to accept a cover since this may cause further injury to the eye if there is something under the eyelid or stuck in the eye.

What You Should Do

First Aid Care for Cut on the Eye or Lid

1. Keep the child in a seated position.

2. Wear disposable gloves.

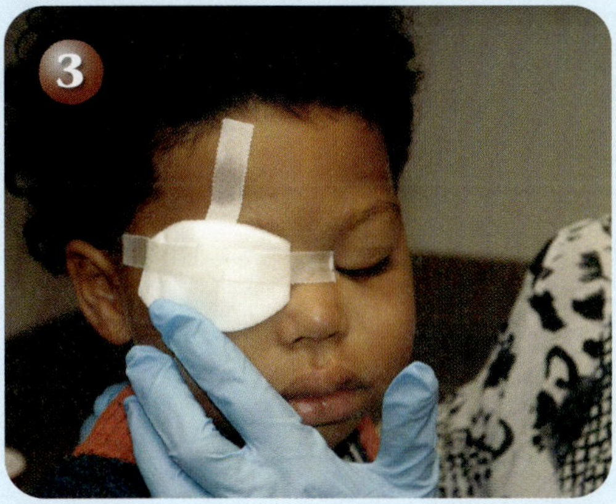

3. If the child will tolerate it, cover the injured eye with a gauze pad and bandage loosely. Do not attempt to flush the eye with water or apply pressure to the injured eyelid. Do not apply medication.

4. Inform the child's parent(s) or legal guardian(s) that the child should be seen by a health care professional.

What You Should Do

First Aid Care for Blow to the Eye

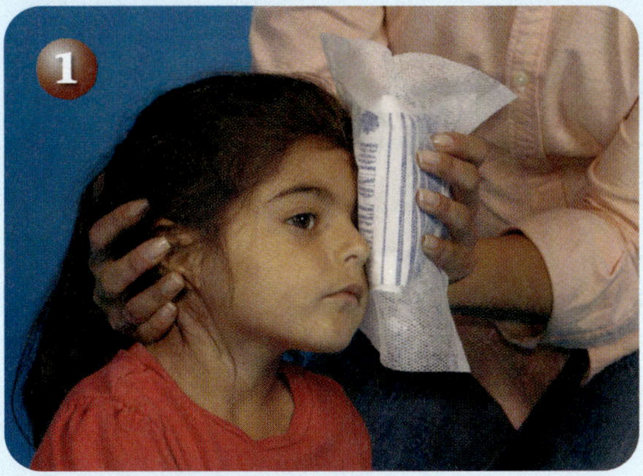

1. Gently place ice pack or a cold pack wrapped in a wet cloth on the injured eye for 10 to 15 minutes to control swelling and reduce pain.

2. A black eye, redness, pain, or blurred vision might indicate internal eye damage or swelling, and the child should be seen by a health care professional as soon as possible. Do not apply medication.

Algorithm

First Aid Care for Chemical in the Eye

Hold injured eye open

↓

Flush with water for 15 minutes

↓

Call poison center

First Aid Care for Penetrating Object in the Eye

Call EMS

↓

Do not remove the object

↓

If object is small, attempt to cover the injured eye with a shield, paper cup, or cardboard folded in a cone over the eye

↓

If the object is long, then place padding around the materials so that it will not dislodge, and bandage the injured eye with a dressing

↓

If accepted by the child, keep child flat on back

First Aid Care for a Foreign Object in the Eye

Pull down the child's lower eye lid

↓

Ask the child to look up. If it is a small speck of dirt, use a wet gauze or handkerchief

↓

Grasp the upper eyelid and pull it out and down over the lower eyelid

↓

If object remains, flush with water

First Aid Care for a Cut on the Eye

Do not apply pressure

↓

If child tolerates it, cover the injured eye with a gauze pad and bandage loosely

Check Your Knowledge

1. Which of the following is not a symptom of an eye injury?
   - a. Double vision
   - b. Sensitivity to light
   - c. Dizziness
   - d. Vomiting and fever
2. If a child gets a chemical in his eye, what is the first thing that you should do?
   - a. Notify the parent(s) or legal guardian(s)
   - b. Fill out an incident report
   - c. Put on disposable gloves and immediately flush the chemical from the eye with lukewarm water
   - d. Call the poison center
3. A corneal abrasion is:
   - a. A scratch of the cornea
   - b. Astigmatism
   - c. When a child loses an eye
   - d. Partial blindness
4. Which of the following is not appropriate care for a child who had something in his eye?
   - a. Pull the upper lid over the lower lid so the tears can dislodge the object
   - b. Let the child rub the eye until it feels better
   - c. Rinse the eye out with clean, running tap water, from the nose side toward the ear side of the eye
   - d. Have someone take the child to a health care professional to manage the problem

Terms

Cornea The transparent outer covering of the eyeball.

Corneal abrasion A scratch of the cornea.

Eye injury Injury to the eye, eyelid, and area around the eye.

Eye trauma Any injury to the eye.

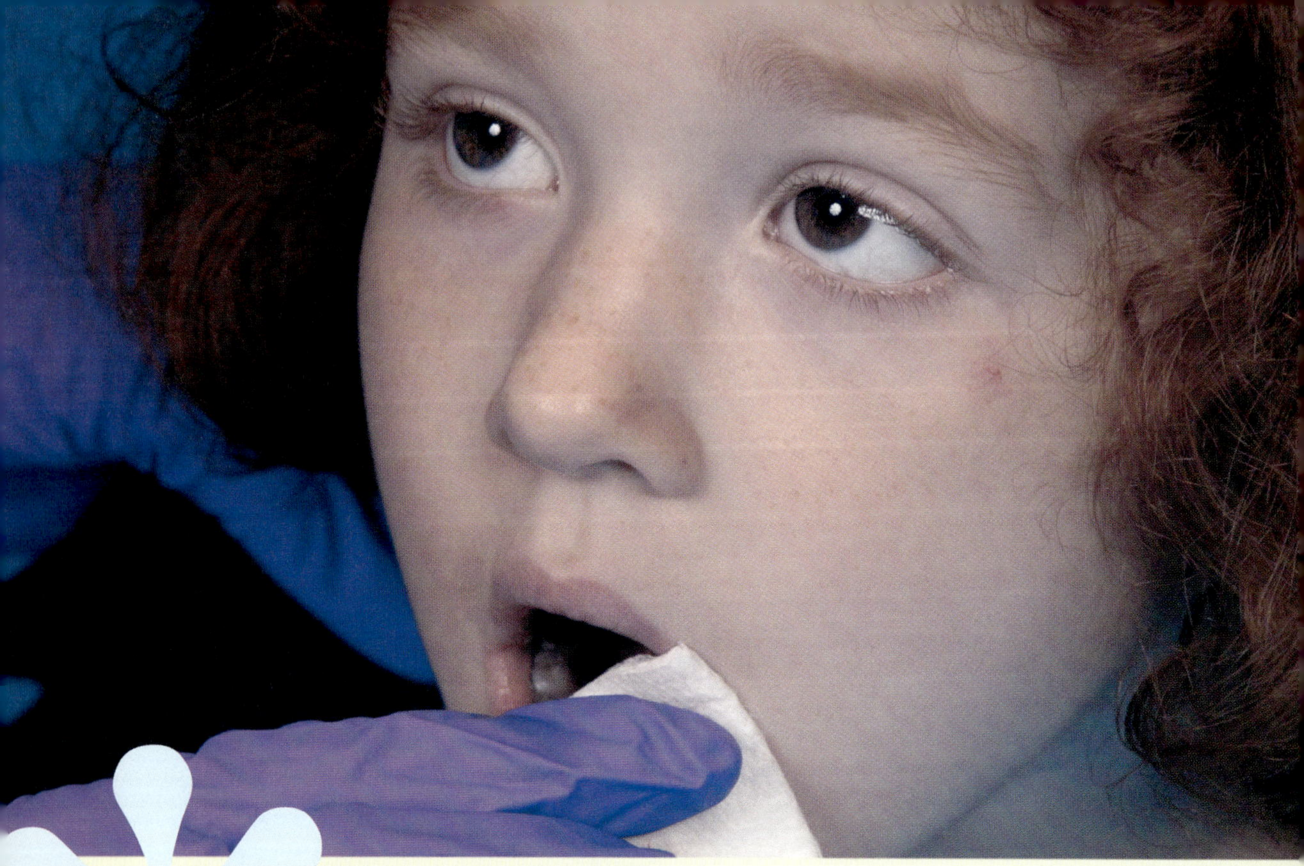

Learning Objectives

The participant will be able to:

- Recognize when a tooth has been knocked out.
- Describe first aid for a knocked-out tooth.
- Describe first aid for a toothache.
- Recognize when a child has a bite to the tongue or lips.
- Describe first aid for a bite to the tongue or lips.

Topic 14

Oral Injuries

Teeth

Introduction

Most children start getting teeth at approximately 6 months of age, and will have a full set of primary, or "baby," teeth by 3 years of age. **Primary teeth** serve a number of purposes. They are involved in speech development, they help maintain good nutrition by allowing the child to chew properly, and they act as space savers for **permanent teeth.** When a child is about 6 years old, his jaw will begin to grow to make room for permanent, or "adult," teeth. From the ages of 6 to 12 years, children will lose primary teeth and permanent teeth will replace them.

What You Should Know

A permanent tooth that is knocked out is a dental emergency that needs immediate first aid. A child with a knocked-out tooth needs to be seen by a dentist as soon as possible. A permanent tooth that is knocked out should be placed back into the socket. This gives the tooth a greater chance of survival. Primary, or baby, teeth should not be reinserted. If a primary tooth is knocked out, the child needs first aid care for any gum injuries and should be seen by a dentist.

What You Should Look For

- A missing tooth in the child's mouth
- Bleeding from the mouth
- Visibly upset child

What You Should Do

The Eight Steps in Pediatric First Aid:

1 Survey the Scene

Take a brief moment to perform a scene survey to ensure that the scene is safe, to find out who is involved, and to determine what happened.

2 Hands-off ABCs

As you approach the child, perform the hands-off ABCs (Appearance, Breathing, and Circulation) to determine if EMS should be called. It should take 15 to 30 seconds or less.

3 Supervise

Immediately ensure that any other children near the scene are properly supervised.

4 Hands-on ABCDEs

Perform the hands-on ABCDEs (Appearance, Breathing, Circulation, Disability, and Everything else) to determine if EMS should be called and what first aid care is needed.

5 First Aid Care

Provide first aid care appropriate to the injury or illness.

6 Notify

As soon as possible, notify the child's parent(s) or legal guardian(s).

7 Debrief

As soon as possible, talk with the child who received first aid about any concerns he or she may have, and talk with other children who witnessed the injury and first aid procedures.

8 Document

Complete an incident report form.

What You Should Do

First Aid Care for Knocked Out Permanent Tooth

1. Position the child so blood does not compromise his airway.
2. Follow Standard Precautions and control any bleeding.

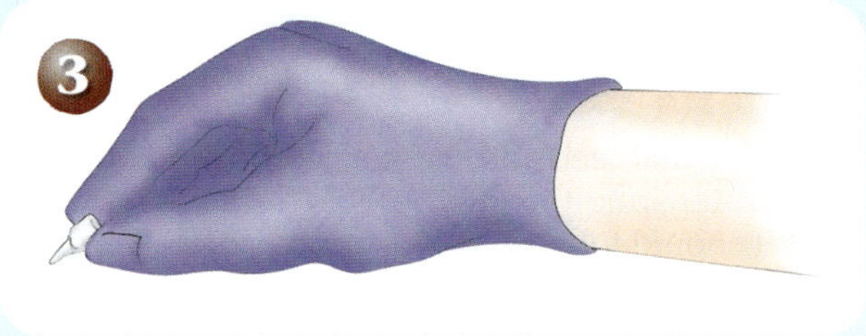

3. Attempt to find the tooth. If you find the tooth, do not handle it by the roots.

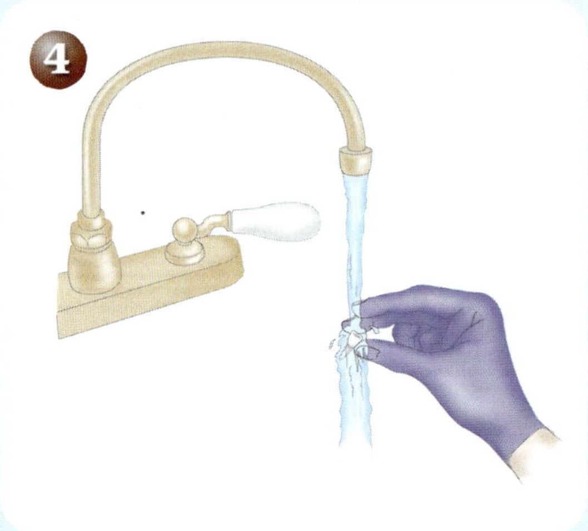

4. If the tooth is dirty, rinse it gently with water. Do not scrub or use antiseptic on the tooth.

First Aid Care for Knocked Out Permanent Tooth (cont.)

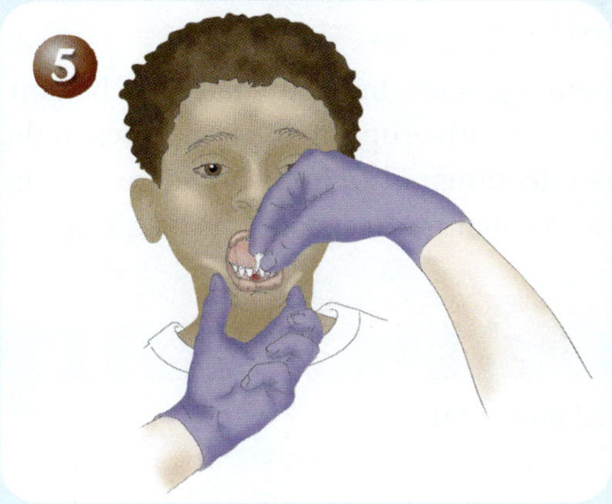

5. Gently place the tooth back in the socket. If the child is able to assist, ask him to hold the tooth in place with a finger or tissue. Do not attempt to reinsert a primary/baby tooth.

6. If the child is upset or resists, or if reinserting the tooth is not possible, place the tooth in a glass of milk. If milk is not available, wrap the tooth in a cold wet cloth.

7. Notify the parent(s) or legal guardian(s) and inform them that the child should be seen by a dentist or health care professional. For best results, the child should be seen by a dentist within one hour of the time the tooth was knocked out.

First Aid Tip

If you are unable to locate a knocked-out tooth, it is still important to have the child seen by a dentist as soon as possible because the tooth may be knocked up into the gums. This is true regardless of whether the tooth is a primary or permanent tooth.

Toothaches

What You Should Know

Toothaches may be dental emergencies, but they may also be confused with discomfort associated with eruption of teeth, sores in the mouth, earaches, and sinus infections. The child should be seen by a dentist or health care professional to determine the origin of the pain or discomfort.

What You Should Look For

- Complaints of pain
- Drooling
- If the child is old enough, ask him to point to what hurts and have him indicate which tooth hurts.

What You Should Do

First Aid Care for Toothaches

1. Follow Standard Precautions.

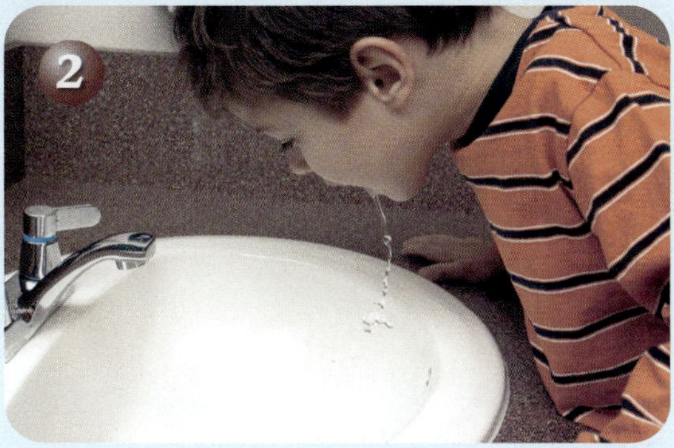

2. Have the child rinse his mouth with warm water.

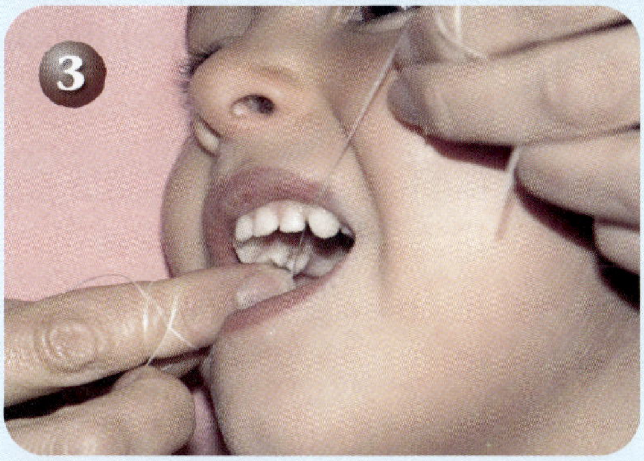

3. Use dental floss to remove any food that might be caught between the teeth.

4. Look for swelling or a "pimple" around the tooth, which may indicate a dental abscess.

5. See if the tooth is loose.

6. Notify the parent(s) or legal guardian(s) and inform them that the child has a toothache and may need to be seen by a dentist or health care professional.

First Aid Tip

If a child complains of a toothache, a pediatrician may be able to identify a problem such as an infection or mouth sores that are giving the child the sensation of a toothache. If these are not the problem, the child needs to be seen by a dentist to determine the cause of the discomfort and to prescribe the proper treatment. If there is any swelling in the mouth or on the face, the child needs to be seen by a health care professional or dentist as soon as possible.

Bites

What You Should Know

Children often bite their lips or tongues while eating or during a fall. A bite to the tongue or lips may be difficult to evaluate because the large amount of bleeding may disguise the true size of the injury.

What to Look For

- A hole in the lip or tongue that is the size and shape of a tooth mark
- Bleeding

What Should You Do

First Aid Care for Bites to the Tongue or Lips

1. Follow Standard Precautions.

2. Have the child rinse with water so that the site of injury can be identified.

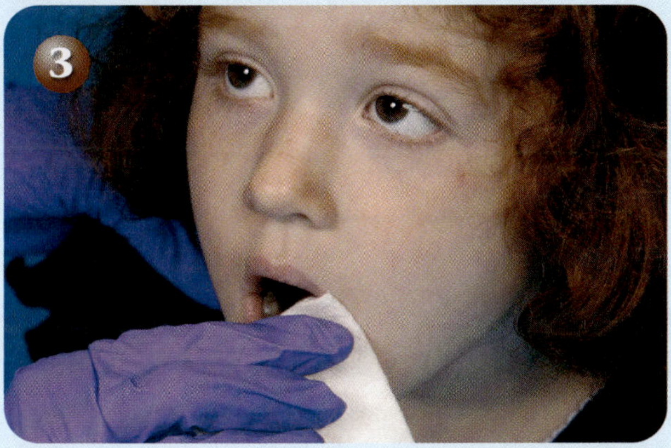

3. Apply pressure with a piece of gauze or cloth to stop the bleeding.

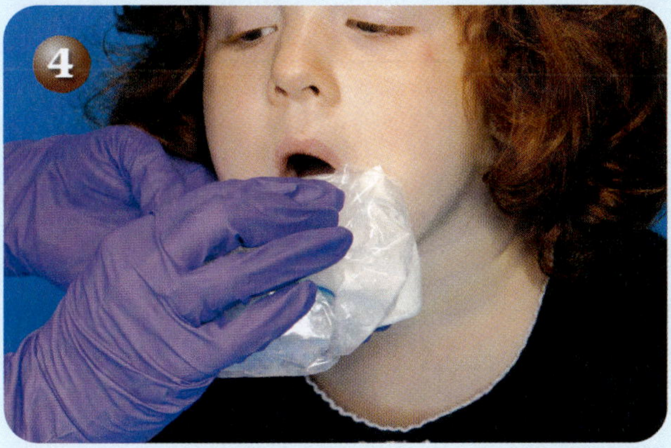

4. Apply ice or a cold pack wrapped in cloth or towel if there is any swelling.

5. Injuries that extend through the lip or that cut across the edge of the tongue should be seen by a health care professional. These injuries may need stitches.

Algorithm

First Aid Care for a Knocked Out Tooth

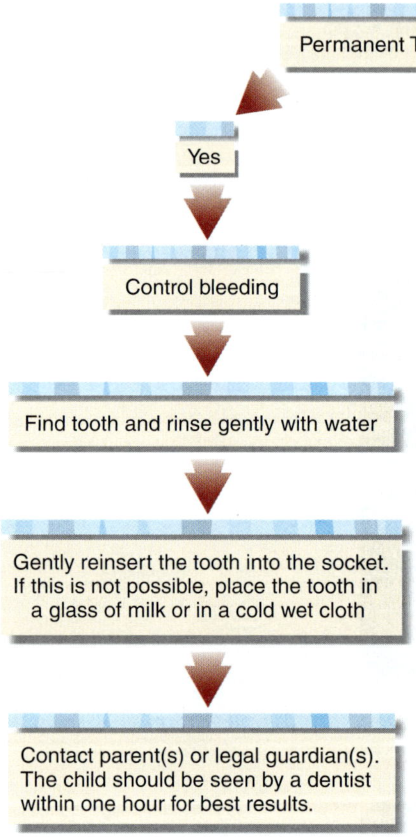

First Aid Care for a Toothache

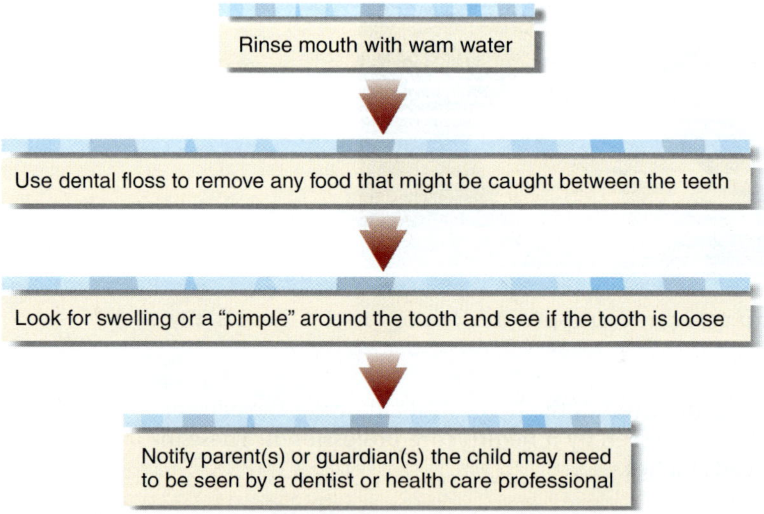

First Aid Care for Lip and Tongue Bites

Have the child rinse with water so that the site of injury can be identified

↓

Apply pressure with a piece of gauze or cloth to stop the bleeding

↓

Apply ice or a cold pack if there is any swelling

↓

Notify the parent(s) or guardian(s)

↓

If the injury extends through the lip into the skin or crosses the edge of the tongue, notify the parent(s) or legal guardian(s). The child should be seen by a health care professional

Check Your Knowledge

Circle the letter next to the response that is the best answer to each question.

1. If a child has had a tooth knocked out, you should:
   a. Reinsert the tooth, regardless of whether it is a permanent tooth or primary tooth
   b. Reinsert only primary teeth
   c. Scrub the tooth and bring the child to the dentist
   d. Attempt to reinsert the tooth only if it is a permanent tooth
2. Most children begin getting teeth at about what age:
   a. 18 months
   b. 14 months
   c. 3 years
   d. 6 months
3. Primary teeth are important for all of the following reasons, except:
   a. They help to maintain good nutrition by enabling proper chewing
   b. They help with speech development
   c. They act as space savers for permanent teeth
   d. They prevent children from choking
4. If a child has a toothache, you should:
   a. Have the child rinse his mouth with warm water
   b. Have someone call the dentist immediately for an appointment
   c. Wiggle or tap on the tooth to see if the pain is from the tooth
   d. Call EMS

Terms

Permanent Teeth Teeth that develop at about 6 years of age to replace primary teeth. By age 21, usually all 32 of the permanent teeth have erupted.

Primary Teeth Also known as baby teeth, primary teeth usually begin to grow at about 6 months of age. Most children have a full set of primary teeth at about age 3.

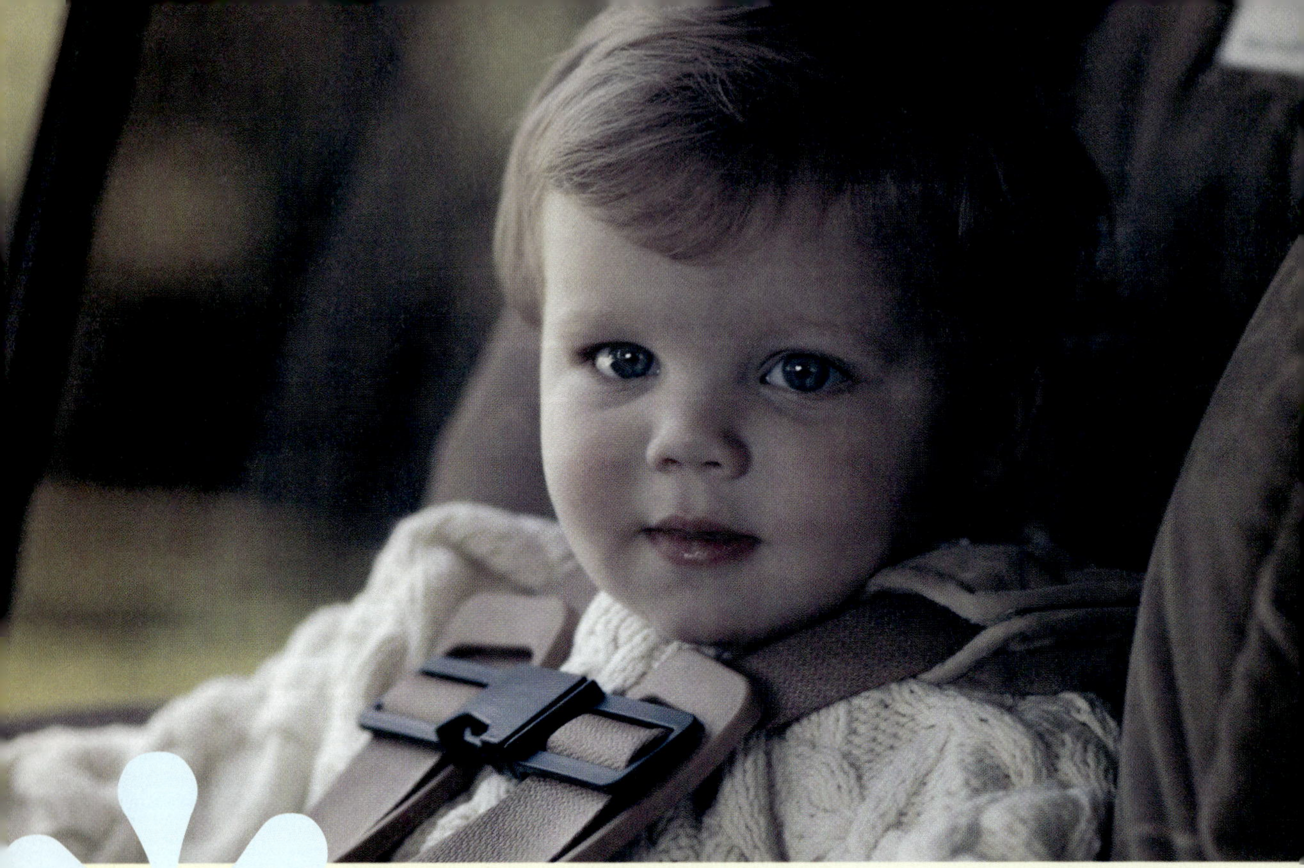

Learning Objectives

The participant will be able to:

- Discuss the importance of prevention in a child care facility.
- List ways to prevent injuries in a child care facility.
- Describe ways to prevent the spread of illnesses in a child care facility.

Topic 15

Prevention

Prevention

Introduction

As a caregiver or teacher, you have the important task of caring and nurturing for young children. In addition to the nurturing aspects of your work, you must also think constantly about the safety of the children. Because children cannot always make judgments about their own health and safety, they tend to be at a greater risk for injuries, such as burns, falls, choking, and poisoning (**Figure 15-1**). Unintentional injuries are often referred to as accidents because they occur unexpectedly and seem uncontrollable. However, most injuries are avoidable if a few simple steps are practiced consistently. **Prevention** is the use of safety measures to reduce risk. In a child care setting, caregivers and teachers should seek to reduce the risk of significant injury or illness to children in their care.

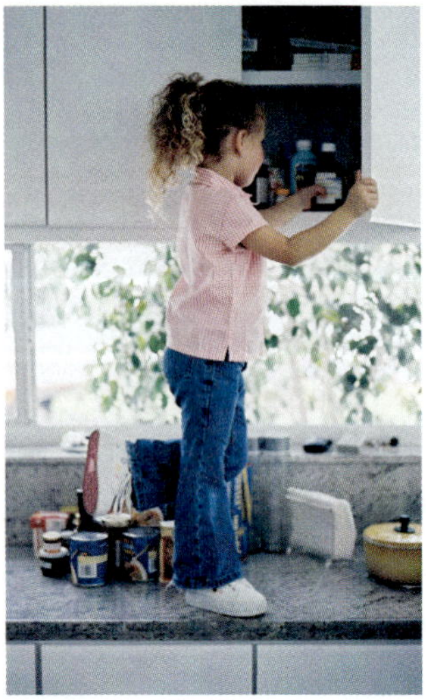

Figure 15-1

Because children cannot always make judgments about their own health and safety, they tend to be at a greater risk for injuries, such as burns, falls, choking, and poisoning.

What You Should Know

Children learn about their environment by exploring; particularly with their senses of taste and touch. Being aware of the dangers in a child's environment and knowing how you can make that environment safer are important in preventing childhood injury and illness. As children grow, the hazards they face change because of their advancing capabilities. Children in a child care setting may be at different ages and developmental stages. This can make creating and maintaining a safe environment particularly challenging. A caregiver or teacher who understands a child's growth and development is invaluable in reducing hazards in the environment with safe age-appropriate items.

Caregivers should seek to maintain child-safe play equipment on playgrounds and in classrooms (**Figure 15-2**). The most common locations for injury in the child care setting are indoor and outdoor play areas. According to the US Consumer Product Safety Commission, National Electronic Injury Surveillance System, each

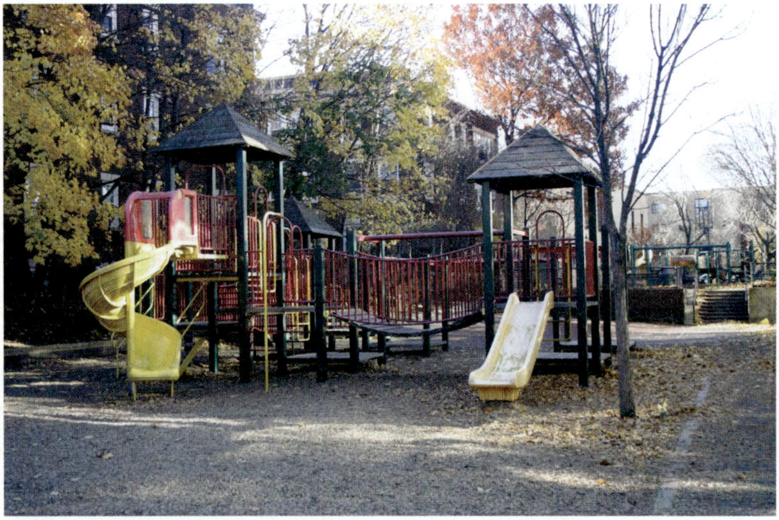

Figure 15-2

Caregivers should seek to maintain child-safe play equipment on playgrounds and in classrooms.

Common Injuries Related to Child's Developmental Level

Developmental Characteristics	Common Injuries
Infant—Age 0 to 1 year	
Increasing mobility	Burns
Uses mouth to explore objects	Choking
Reaches for and pulls objects	Drowning
Unaware of dangers	Falls
Cannot understand "no"	
Toddler—Age 1 to 2½ years	
Travels in cars	Burns
Masters walking, running, climbing	Choking
Explores almost everything with mouth	Drowning
Begins to imitate behaviors	Falls
Investigates everything within reach	Motor vehicle passenger and pedestrian injuries
Curious about never-before-seen items	Poisoning
Unaware of most dangers	Suffocation
Impulsive	
Preschooler—Age 2½ to 5 years	
Travels in cars	Burns
Mobility leads to increased independence	Choking
Learns to ride tricycle	Drowning
Unaware of many dangers	Falls
Might favor real tools, gadgets, appliances rather than toys	Motor vehicle passenger and pedestrian injuries
Fascinated with fire	Poisoning
Imitates adult behavior	
School-aged—Age 5 years and up	
Travels in cars	Bicycle injuries
Walks alone	Burns
Seeks independence	Falls
Wants to be like peers	Firearm injuries
Likes to be with peers	Motor vehicle passenger and pedestrian injuries
Needs increased physical activity	
Dangers do not always seem real	
Increased independence can mean less supervision	

year approximately 200,000 US children aged 14 years and under pay a visit to the emergency department as a result of injuries received on the playground. Most of the playground injuries occur when a child falls, collides with equipment, or catches his clothes or a part of his body on the equipment. Playground equipment that poses the highest risk include monkey bars, ladders, swings, and climbers. Items used in the facility should be warranted by the manufacturer and installer to meet the standards of the Consumer Product Safety Commission (CPSC) and the American Society for Testing and Materials (ASTM).

What You Should Look For

Identifying potential dangers is an initial step in creating a safe environment. The first thing that you can do to recognize potential danger is to conduct a child's eye-level inspection in every room of the child care facility. For example, look for electrical outlets that do not have protective covers on them to prevent access by children and any cleaning supplies or household products that could be within a child's reach. Check that all hanging cords, table coverings, and lamps are out of reach and cannot be pulled on by a child. Are the medicine cabinets locked and the doors that lead to stairways, outdoors, and storage areas properly secured? Check all indoor and outdoor equipment that is accessible to children. Is the equipment well-maintained and appropriate for the developmental level of the children? Creative use of play areas and thoughtful storage of toys may be required.

Each day before children arrive at the facility, a caregiver or teacher should take a quick walk around the facility to make sure that the facility is safe and clean. Learning and following the prevention measures outlined in "What You Should Do" will help you to recognize potential dangers in your facility.

First Aid Tip

It is important that child care providers have, and are prepared to follow, a care plan for any child with a special health care need. Caregivers also need access to a telephone and emergency contact numbers for each child in the facility. This should be accessible both in the facility and during any type of off-site trip.

What You Should Do

Prevention steps can reduce the likelihood that you will need to use your first aid skills. However, if a first aid emergency occurs, it is important to follow the eight steps of pediatric first aid.

The Eight Steps in Pediatric First Aid:

1 Survey the Scene

Take a brief moment to perform a scene survey to ensure that the scene is safe, to find out who is involved, and to determine what happened.

2 Hands-off ABCs

As you approach the child, perform the hands-off ABCs (Appearance, Breathing, and Circulation) to determine if EMS should be called. It should take 15 to 30 seconds or less.

3 Supervise

Immediately ensure that any other children near the scene are properly supervised.

4 Hands-on ABCDEs

Perform the hands-on ABCDEs (Appearance, Breathing, Circulation, Disability, and Everything else) to determine if EMS should be called and what first aid care is needed.

5 First Aid Care

Provide first aid care appropriate to the injury or illness.

6 Notify

As soon as possible, notify the child's parent(s) or legal guardian(s).

7 Debrief

As soon as possible, talk with the child who received first aid about any concerns he or she may have and also talk with other children who have witnessed the injury and first aid procedures.

8 Document

Complete an incident report form.

What You Should Do

Prevention of Injuries

- Any stairway, window, balcony, or elevated surface that is used by or accessible to the children in the facility should be properly secured and meet ASTM standards.
- Remove sharp-edged furniture.
- Do not use baby walkers that can move across the floor. A baby may tip the walker over, fall out of it, or fall down stairs and seriously injure his head. Baby walkers let children get to places where they can pull heavy objects or hot food on themselves.
- Do not leave a baby alone on changing tables, beds, sofas, or chairs.
- Lock the doors to any potentially dangerous areas.
- Use gates or doors on stairways and doorways.
- Operable window guards should be installed on all windows above the first floor.
- The surface under play equipment should be made of a cushioning material rated to absorb the force of a fall. A manufactured and height-rated rubber mat, or at least 12 inches of sand, sawdust, or wood chips underneath play equipment should be used.

What You Should Do

Prevention of the Spread of Illnesses

Controlling Bleeding (on page 43) details information about Universal and Standard Precautions. To prevent infection and the spread of illness:

- Reduce contact with germs.
- Use barriers, such as non-porous gloves, disposable diaper table papers, disposable towels for cleaning-up and sanitizing surfaces, non-porous surfaces that can be cleaned and sanitized, and plastic bags to store contaminated articles until they can be thrown away or sanitized.

- Use whatever tools (e.g., paper towels, tissues, rags, and mops) you have to wipe up any spilled body fluid. Try to use disposable tools to minimize the need to do further cleaning and sanitizing. Avoid spreading spilled body fluid around.
- Put all tools (e.g., paper towels, tissues, rags, mops) that you used to wipe up the spill into a plastic-lined receptacle for disposal or to clean and sanitize later.
- Use a detergent to clean all surfaces in contact with the spill, including floors and rugs.
- Rinse cleaned surfaces with water.
- Apply a sanitizing solution, following the manufacturer's instructions on the label.
- Put body fluid contaminated material used to clean and sanitize the surfaces in a plastic bag with a secure tie for disposal.
- For additional suggestions on cleaning, sanitizing, and preventing spread of illness, refer to *Caring for Our Children: National Health and Safety Performance Standards: Guidelines for Out-of-Home Child Care Programs, Second Edition.*

What You Should Do

Prevention of Choking

- Supervise mealtime.
- Insist that children sit down while eating. Children should never run, walk, play, or lie down with food in their mouths.
- Cut food for infants and young children into pieces no larger than ½ inch.
- Encourage children to chew their food well.
- Be aware of older children's actions. Many choking incidents occur when an older child gives a dangerous food, toy, or small object to a younger child.
- Keep the following foods away from children under 4 years of age:
  - Hot dogs
  - Nuts and seeds
  - Chunks of meat or cheese
  - Whole grapes

  - Hard or sticky candy
  - Popcorn
  - Chunks of peanut butter
  - Chunks of raw vegetables
  - Chewing gum
- Avoid toys with small parts and keep other small household items out of the reach of infants and young children.
- Follow the age recommendations on toy packages. Age guidelines reflect the safety of a toy based on any possible choking hazard as well as the child's physical and mental abilities at various ages.
- Check under furniture and between cushions for small items that children could find and put in their mouths.
- Other items that can be choking hazards and should be kept away from infants and young children, include:
  - Latex balloons
  - Coins
  - Marbles
  - Toys with small parts
  - Toys that can be compressed to fit entirely into a child's mouth
  - Small balls
  - Pen or marker caps
  - Small button-type batteries

What You Should Do

Prevention of Burns

- The water temperature and all hot surfaces accessible to children at the facility should not exceed 120°F.
- Keep cribs, cots, and beds at a safe distance from radiators and electrical outlets.
- Cover outlets with special child-resistant face plates or other safety devices. Plastic plug covers can be a choking hazard if loose-fitting or when removed to use the outlet.

- Do not allow electrical cords to dangle over the edge of countertops.
- Regularly check for frayed or damaged electrical cords.
- Do not use extension cords around infants and toddlers. A child can be electrocuted by biting through a live electric cord.
- Do not run electric cords under rugs in areas of heavy traffic.
- Do not overload electrical circuits.
- Teach children that fire burns.
- Keep matches and lighters out of the reach of children.
- All smoke detectors should be tested and working properly.
- Have a fire escape plan with a designated place for all the children and adults to go. Hold practice fire drills regularly.
- Fire extinguishers should be kept in accessible locations.

What You Should Do

Prevention of Bites and Stings

- When walking in tall grasses, woods, or fields, children's legs should be covered. If possible, tuck pants into socks and long-sleeved shirts at the waist and have the children wear sneakers instead of sandals.
- Stay on trails whenever possible.
- Check children's skin after playing in these areas. Pay special attention to the folds of the skin, the scalp, and the back of the neck. Removing a tick within the first 24 hours greatly reduces the risk of infection.
- Contact your local health department to find out if deer ticks are prevalent in your area.
- Spray insect repellent only when outdoors, use sparingly, and wash hands after applying. Never apply insect repellent to the face, to an open wound, or cut, or to the hands or arms of a child who is likely to put sprayed skin in his mouth.
- Report any insect nests or hives that pose a risk to the children around the facility to the appropriate personnel for removal.
- Check for nests in other locations where children play such as in old tree stumps or playground equipment.

- Avoid garbage cans and dumpsters.
- When eating outdoors, be aware that many foods attract insects, especially: tuna, peanut butter and jelly sandwiches, watermelon, sweetened beverages, and ice cream.

What You Should Do

Prevention of Poisoning

- Limit use of toxic substances as much as possible. For pest control, use the Integrated Pest Management (IPM) approach that involves sealing up openings that allow pests to enter, putting food in pest-resistant containers, and selecting least-toxic pest control chemicals.
- Eliminate careless storage of poisonous substances. Keep all chemical substances out of reach of children, including household products. Store products in locked cabinets or on high, secure shelves.
- Lock medicine cabinets.
- Avoid interruptions when using a poisonous product.
- Do not store household products with food; the differences between them may not be apparent to a young child.
- Whenever possible, use products with child-resistant safety caps. Remember that, although these are much safer than standard containers, they are not completely childproof. Children watch and imitate adult behavior, and some children can master the skill of opening the lids. Also, if the lids are not completely closed, they will not be child resistant.
- Keep products in their original, labeled containers. If a poisonous substance is swallowed, correct identification is critical for proper treatment. Do not reuse empty containers such as juice bottles to store chemicals.
- Remember that nonprescription medicines can be just as dangerous as prescription medicines.
- Give prescription medicine only to the child for whom it is intended. What can help one child can harm another.

- Check the medicine label for the dosage each time you administer medication. Use a dose-measuring cup or spoon. More is not better when giving medicine.
- Never call medicine "candy."
- In areas accessible to children, identify and remove indoor and outdoor plants at your center that may be toxic if eaten.

What You Should Do

Prevention of Heat and Cold Related Injuries

Heat

- Encourage children to drink cool water frequently.
- Avoid vigorous physical activity during the mid-day hours when temperatures are usually the highest.
- Encourage parent(s) and legal guardian(s) to dress children in lightweight and loose-fitting, sun protective clothing in hot weather.
- Never leave a child in a closed vehicle without an adult in the vehicle to directly supervise the child.

Cold

- Wearing dry mittens, hats, insulated and water-repellent boots and snow pants, and other attire may help to prevent cold injuries.
- Bring a child indoors immediately if he complains of a cold, numb, tingling, or painful area on the body.

What You Should Do

Prevention of Sudden Infant Death Syndrome (SIDS)

Sudden Infant Death Syndrome (SIDS) is described as an unexplained death in infants under 1 year of age. The death is not attributed to any medical condition or external factor, such as abuse or neglect, but is an unexplainable condition with no known preventable causes.

Recommendations to reduce the risk of SIDS are:

- Place infants on their backs when sleeping; utilize a device specially designed to keep babies from rolling over onto their stomachs.
- Do not smoke around or take infants to smoky establishments.
- Avoid overheating the baby with blankets or heaters.

It is important to remember that if the infant is warm and not breathing rescue attempts should not be delayed. Do not waste time, begin rescue breathing immediately, then activate EMS.

What You Should Do

Prevention of Other Injuries

Think ahead whenever possible. Consider what could happen if a child was able to get to whatever is in the environment. While making the environment risk-free is not possible, the goal is to avoid situations that are likely to lead to serious injury.

What You Should Do

In Case of a Catastrophic Emergency

- There should be at least one readily available first aid kit wherever children are in care. This includes one for field trips and outings away from the facility and one to remain at the facility. A first aid kit should also be kept in each vehicle that is used to transport children to and from child care. The first aid kits should contain:
  - Disposable nonporous gloves
  - Scissors
  - Tweezers

- A nonglass thermometer
- Bandage tape
- Sterile gauze pads
- Flexible roller gauze
- Triangular bandages
- Safety pins
- Eye dressing
- Pen/pencil and notepad
- Cold pack
- Current American Academy of Pediatrics' 3-in-1 First Aid, Choking, CPR Chart, or equivalent first aid guide
- Flashlight
- Whistle
- Battery-powered radio
- Water (1 gallon per person per day)
- Emergency food (three-day supply of non-perishable food)
- Can opener
- Liquid soap
- Moist towelettes, garbage bags, and plastic ties
- Adhesive strip bandages, plastic bags for cloths, gauze, and other materials used in handling bodily fluids
- Any emergency medications and medical information needed for children with special needs
- List of emergency phone numbers, phone numbers for parents and legal guardians, and the poison control center number

Check Your Knowledge

1. Which of the following are not considered developmental characteristics in infants?

   a. Do not understand the word, "No"

   b. Are unaware of dangers

   c. Have increasing mobility

   d. Imitate adult behavior

2. All of the following are potential choking hazards, except:

   a. Hot dogs

   b. Whole grapes

   c. Popcorn

   d. Applesauce

3. Prevention:

   a. Is the use of safety measures to minimize risk.

   b. Teaches people how to care for an open wound.

   c. Means there is no longer any risks in the environment.

   d. Stops any accidents from occurring.

4. Barriers that are used to prevent the spread of infection and the spread of illness, include all of the following except:

   a. Non-porous gloves

   b. Disposable towels

   c. Plastic bags

   d. Ointment

Terms

Prevention The use of safety measures to minimize potential risk.

Appendices

A: Common Childhood Illnesses

B: American Academy of Pediatrics 3-in-1 First Aid, Choking, CPR Chart

Anal Itching

Possible Causes: Pinworms, inadequate toilet hygiene, tight underwear or pants

What You Should Know

Pinworms are caused by an intestinal parasitic worm. An infection is acquired by ingesting microscopic pinworm eggs. It is common among young children who often put their hands in their mouths and who are poor hand washers. Many children have pinworms without noticeable symptoms. It is highly contagious in a family or childcare setting, because it spreads to others when the child scratches the anal area, gets eggs under the fingernails, and then touches another child's food or other items that might be put in the mouth. It also spreads from eggs on pajamas, linens, underpants, and so on.

Pinworm can be diagnosed with a special pinworm kit used by the parent to collect specimens from the anal skin. Note: that the "kit" is not available over the counter. A simple test is the "Scotch® tape test." Parents apply Scotch® tape to their child's anus (rectum) first thing in the morning to collect any small threadlike white pinworms. The tape is removed and another piece of tape is placed over it to seal it. The specimen can then be taken to the doctor, or their doctor may have them bring it to a hospital laboratory.

Poor toilet hygiene is common among young children. When girls do not wipe after urinating, and boys or girls do not wipe well after a bowel movement, the skin in the area that is damp or soiled may become irritated, causing itching.

If clothing worn over the anal area is too small, it may irritate the child and cause the child to frequently clutch and pull at the clothing.

What You Should Look For

- Itching and irritation around the anal or vaginal area
- Irritated or soiled skin and underpants
- Clutching at underwear, shorts, tights, or pants

What You Should Do

Caregivers and parents should

1. Discourage scratching of the anal area.
2. Encourage the child to wash hands after using the toilet and before touching food or anything that goes into the mouth.
3. Encourage girls to dry the vaginal area after urinating and both boys and girls to wipe feces off the skin after bowel movements (wiping front to back).
4. Check whether underwear, tights, shorts, or pants are too small for comfort.
5. If pinworms are the problem, seek advice about treatment from the child's primary care provider. Wash and sanitize toys and surfaces used for eating, toileting, hand washing, food preparation, and diapering whenever they are likely to have been soiled.

Caregivers should

1. Notify the child's parents.
2. Discuss possible causes for the problem with the parents.
3. If pinworms are the problem, suggest that staff and family members watch for symptoms in others who have been exposed.

Parents should

1. Consult the child's primary care provider for testing and treatment.
2. Follow caregiver recommendations.

3. Trim the child's fingernails short.
4. Wash child's bed linen, clothing, and towels in hot water and dry on the high heat setting; do not shake items, because this will scatter the eggs.

Child May Return to School or Child Care . . .

Children do not need to be excluded from school or child care for anal itching, even if the symptoms are caused by pinworms.

Constipation

What You Should Know

Constipation is defined as hard stools that cause painful elimination. It can be caused by a diet low in fiber and inadequate fluid intake. Sometimes it may result from postponing or resisting the urge to eliminate.

What You Should Look For

- Many days without normal bowel movements
- Hard stools that are difficult or painful to pass, or stools that are unusually large or hard to flush down the toilet
- Abdominal pain (stomachaches, cramping, nausea)
- Rectal bleeding from tears called fissures
- Fecal soiling of underwear in a child who has learned to use the toilet
- Poor appetite
- Cranky behavior

What You Should Do

Caregivers and parents should

1. Encourage child to drink enough clear fluids to keep the child's urine pale colored.
2. Encourage child to eat foods that contain fiber and have a tendency to soften the stool, such as whole-grain products, peaches, prunes, grapes, raisins, plums, melons, carrots, celery, and lettuce.
3. Reduce intake of foods that bind, such as milk, hard cheese, cottage cheese, bananas, apples, applesauce, and white-flour baked goods.
4. Encourage regular toileting at times when typically a child might need to have a stool. For most people, the urge to have a bowel movement comes after eating or exercising.

Caregivers should

Notify parents.

Parents should

1. Work with the child's caregiver to set regular times for the child to have a relaxed opportunity to use the toilet when the child is most likely to feel the urge to have a bowel movement—usually after meals or after exercise.
2. Call child's health care provider if problem persists for several weeks, or sooner if the child develops vomiting or a large abdomen (belly).

Child May Return to School or Child Care . . .

The child need not be excluded from school or child care.

Coughing

What You Should Know

Coughing is a symptom of an irritation anywhere within the respiratory tract. It often accompanies a viral infection such as a cold. Also, coughing may be caused by an ear infection, allergy, asthma, croup, or infection in any part of the body involved in breathing.

What You Should Look For

- Sore throat
- Dry or wet cough
- Throat irritation
- Hoarse voice, barking cough

What You Should Do

Caregivers and parents should

1. Teach children to cover their mouths when coughing with a disposable facial tissue if possible or with a shoulder if no facial tissue is available in time.
2. Wash hands thoroughly and often.
3. Watch for difficulty breathing.

Caregivers should:

Notify parents.

Parents should

1. Follow caregiver recommendations.
2. Notify child's health care provider if child develops a fever, has trouble catching his or her breath, or if cough persists for longer than 1 week.

Child May Return to School or Child Care . . .

Child need not be excluded from school or child care unless the cough is severe or the child has difficulty breathing.

A Possible Cause of Coughing: Pertussis (Whooping Cough)

What You Should Know

Pertussis is commonly known as "whooping cough" because of the whooping noise a child makes when coughing. It is a highly contagious bacterial infection that spreads to others through coughing and sneezing. The incubation period averages 7 to 10 days, with a range of 5 to 21 days. It is generally a mild illness in older children, but it can be life threatening to infants because of breathing difficulties and the risk of pneumonia.

Pertussis is diagnosed by nasal culture. It is treated with antibiotics for 14 to 21 days. A vaccine is given to infants as part of the DPT (diptheria, pertussis, tetanus) immunization to protect young children, but immunity takes multiple doses of vaccine, with boosters to maintain protection.

What You Should Look For

- Begins with coldlike signs or symptoms
- Coughing that may progress to severe coughing, which may cause vomiting, loss of breath, difficulty catching breath, and blueness of skin
- Whooping sound when inhaling after a period of coughing
- Absent or minimal fever

What You Should Do

Caregivers and parents should

1. Report to local health authorities.
2. Ensure that all children have received their immunization series according to current recommendations.
3. Monitor staff and children for respiratory signs or symptoms for 21 days after the last contact with an infected child.

Caregivers should

1. Encourage parents of a child with a prolonged cough to take the child to a health care provider.
2. Alert other parents if their children have been exposed to a child who is diagnosed with pertussis. Encourage them to contact their health care providers. Maintain confidentiality.
3. Monitor staff for respiratory illness and recommend that they seek treatment if they develop a persistent cough.

Parents should

Have the child seen by a health care provider for prolonged cough.

Child May Return to School or Child Care . . .

The child may return to school or child care after 5 days of appropriate antimicrobial therapy, which must be continued for the total number of days prescribed. Depending on the antibiotic used, the total treatment time can be 5–14 days.

Diaper Rash

Possible Cause: Simple Diaper Rash

What You Should Know

Diaper rash commonly occurs when surfaces that are wet by urine or stool rub against the skin. Also, bacteria in the bowel react with urine to form ammonia, which may irritate and burn skin. Diaper rash can be painful.

What You Should Look For

- Redness
- Raw skin
- Red bumps
- Sores
- Cracking of skin in the diaper region

What You Should Do

Caregivers and parents should

1. Use commercially available disposable diapers with absorbent material that keeps the surface of the diaper that touches the child dry.
2. Change diapers often—checking hourly by the look, feel, or smell of the diapers through clothing, and by opening the diaper to look for wetness or feces at least every 2 hours.
3. Wash diaper area with soap and warm water; allow to dry completely.
4. Place child in cool baths with one-half cup vinegar for 15 to 20 minutes several times per day. Vinegar reduces bacterial growth and helps to neutralize ammonia.

5. Protect diaper area with over-the-counter ointments, such as zinc oxide or petroleum jelly, which act as moisture barriers.
6. Wash hands thoroughly after removing soiled diapers and clothing, even if gloves have been used during the changing.
7. Baby powder or cornstarch are not recommended.
8. If cloth diapers are being used, they should be of the type that includes an absorbent inner lining completely contained within an outer covering made of a waterproof material so that the outer covering and inner lining are changed together as a unit. The liner and diaper should be removed when soiled, and then cleaned, disinfected, washed, rinsed, and dried or chemically disinfected. Rinsing in a dilute solution of vinegar may help to remove any residual detergent or other chemicals that might irritate the child's skin.

Caregivers should

Notify parents.

Parents should

Follow caregiver recommendations.

Child May Return to School or Child Care . . .

The child need not be excluded from school or child care.

Possible Cause: Candida Diaper Infection

What You Should Know

Candida is a type of yeast that lives within the intestines of healthy people. It can infect moist areas of skin. It is treated with prescription medication. For additional information, see Thrush on page 277.

What You Should Look For

Appears as a fiery red rash.

What You Should Do

Caregivers and parents should

1. Change diapers often.
2. Clean the skin in the diaper area carefully and then dry the area completely.
3. Apply a thin layer of any cream that has been prescribed to the affected skin.
4. Wash hands thoroughly after completing the diapering routine.

Caregivers should

1. Wash and sanitize diaper changing areas after each diaper change.
2. Keep child's skin clean and dry.
3. Notify parents.

Parents should

1. Follow caregiver recommendations.
2. Call child's health care provider for prescription medication.

Child May Return to School or Child Care . . .

Exclusion of children who have a diaper rash is not required.

Diarrhea

What You Should Know

Diarrhea is watery stools, less-formed stools than usual, and more frequent stools. It is caused primarily by viruses. It also can be caused by bacterial or parasitic infections, some medications (especially antibiotics), changes in diet, and certain foods. It may resolve without treatment within a few days. If mild diarrhea does not resolve within a few days or if there is blood in the diarrhea, the child should be seen by a health care provider for a stool culture to determine if the diarrhea is infectious.

What You Should Look For

- Frequent loose or watery stools compared to the child's normal pattern
- Abdominal cramps
- Fever
- Generally not feeling well
- Blood in the stool

What You Should Do

Caregivers and parents should

1. Not let children and adults who have diarrhea handle food.
2. Call a health care professional if the child has any of the following:
   - Blood in stool
   - Frequent vomiting
   - Abdominal pain
   - Less frequent urination
   - No tears when crying

- Loss of appetite for liquids
- High fever
- Frequent or persistent diarrhea
- Dry, sticky mouth
- Weight loss
- Extreme thirst

Caregivers should

1. Notify parents.
2. Practice particularly careful and frequent hand washing, especially after using the toilet or handling soiled diapers, and before anything having to do with food preparation or eating.
3. Exclude children with diarrhea who cannot use the toilet for all bowel movements. This means exclusion of all infants and children in diapers with diarrhea and all children who use the toilet but are having "accidents" when they do not use the toilet for stool.

Parents should

Follow caregiver recommendations.

Child May Return to School or Child Care . . .

- If cleared by a health professional after bloody diarrhea and diarrhea caused by certain bacteria (e.g., *Shigella, Salmonella, E. Coli* 0157:H7) or the parasite *Giardia lamblia.*
- When stool is contained in the toilet (for toilet-trained children).
- Even if stools stay loose, the child may return when the child seems well and the stool consistency has not changed for a week.
- When the child can participate in the program and the staff determine that they can care for the child without compromising their ability to care for the other children in the group.

Possible Problem: *Escherichia coli* diarrhea

What You Should Know

Many types of *E. coli* bacteria live normally in the intestine; however, at least five types are known to cause diarrhea. Two types have caused numerous outbreaks in group care settings. Infections with *E. coli* O157:H7 may be associated with other severe problems, such as bleeding from irritation of the bowel, kidney damage, and blood cell damage. The incubation period ranges from 1 to 8 days, and the child is contagious until the diarrhea resolves and test results come back negative twice.

E. coli is spread through direct contact with infected people or eating contaminated food or water (undercooked ground beef, unpasteurized milk, apple cider, raw vegetables, salami, yogurt, untreated drinking water in recreation areas). It can be prevented by cooking all ground beef so there is no pink meat and only using pasteurized products.

What You Should Look For

- Loose stools, which may be watery and bloody
- Abdominal pain
- Fever

What You Should Do

Caregivers and parents should

1. Notify health professionals.
2. Wash hands often.

Caregivers should

Notify parents.

Parents should

1. Notify health professionals.
2. Wash hands often.

Child May Return to School or Child Care . . .

When health professionals give approval.

Possible Problem: Infectious Diarrhea

What You Should Know

Infectious diarrhea varies from mild to severe and is highly contagious. It is acquired by ingestion of contaminated water or food. It is an intestinal infection caused by viruses or by bacteria such as *Salmonella* and *Shigella* species, a parasite such as *Giardia lamblia,* or a virus. Bacterial or parasitic infections and some viral infections of the intestine can be diagnosed by stool culture(s). Some bacterial infections are treated with prescription medication, but others require that the body rid itself of the infection.

What You Should Look For

- Diarrhea containing blood or mucus
- Stomach or abdominal cramping and gas
- Foul-smelling stools
- Fever
- Weight loss

What You Should Do

Caregivers and parents should

1. Encourage child to drink extra amounts of clear fluids, but not fruit juices.
2. Do not allow child to share drinking glasses or eating utensils with others.

Caregivers should

1. Wear disposable gloves for diapering or helping with toileting to reduce chances of spreading infection. Wash hands thoroughly after removing gloves.
2. Notify parents.

Parents should

1. Follow caregiver recommendations.
2. Contact child's health care provider for instructions for treatment and prevention of spread to other family members.

Child May Return to School or Child Care . . .

- When the specific recommended treatment and laboratory testing required for the type of infection has been completed. *Note:* Salmonella is not always treated. Medication may prolong the carrier state. Children who have no symptoms but have *Giarda lamblia* in their stools do not need to be excluded from child care or school.
- In all cases, check with your health care provider about a child's return after the child has been excluded for infectious diarrhea with a positive laboratory test.

Possible Problem: Hepatitis A

What You Should Know

Hepatitis A is a viral infection that causes inflammation of the liver. It enters the body via the mouth and spreads through contact with stool. Infected children do not necessarily have any recognizable symptoms, but infected adults can be very sick. It does not usually cause diarrhea. Instead, it causes loss of appetite, nausea, jaundice (yellowing of the skin and whites of the eyes), fever, fatigue, and brown urine. It spreads from person to person when hands contaminated with microscopic particles of stool touch food or eating utensils. People who have the infection are most contagious for 2 weeks before signs or symptoms develop, but the infection can be in the incubation (developing) stage for 1 to 2 months before there are any symptoms. Those who have hepatitis A stop spreading the disease about a week after the jaundice develops.

What You Should Look For

- Fever
- Jaundice (yellowing of skin or whites of eyes)
- Abdominal discomfort
- Tiredness
- Dark-brown urine
- Loss of appetite
- Nausea

What You Should Do

Caregivers and parents should

1. Prevent the disease by getting the hepatitis A vaccine.
2. If you are exposed to someone with hepatitis A or suspect that the disease is developing, contact your health care provider immediately.

3. Do not allow child to share drinking glasses or eating utensils with others.

Caregivers should

1. Wear disposable gloves for diapering or helping with toileting to reduce chances of spreading infection. Remove gloves after disposing of soiled clothing and before putting on clean undergarments. Wipe hands with a disposable wipe immediately after removing gloves and then wash hands thoroughly as the last step in the diapering or toileting process.
2. Inform parents.
3. Contact your health care provider if you are exposed to the hepatitis A virus.

Parents should

1. Follow caregiver recommendations.
2. Contact the child's health care provider if any family member is exposed to the hepatitis A virus.

Child May Return to School or Child Care . . .

- Child should remain at home for 1 week after developing symptoms.
- Check with your health care provider concerning protection of others who may have been exposed to hepatitis A infection.

Possible Problem: Rotavirus

What You Should Know

Rotavirus is a virus that belongs to a family of viruses found worldwide. It is one of the most common causes of diarrhea and vomiting, especially from late fall to early spring. It is the single most common cause of diarrhea in children younger than 2 years. Rotavirus can cause serious illness in infants and toddlers. Nearly all children have been infected with it by age 3. Children can become infected more than once because the virus has many types. The incubation period is 2 to 4 days, and the child is contagious up to 3 weeks after the illness. It is spread through the fecal-oral route.

What You Should Look For

- Nonbloody diarrhea
- Nausea
- Vomiting
- Dehydration in severe cases
- Generally lasts 3 to 8 days

What You Should Do

Caregivers and parents should

1. Routinely practice proper hand washing, especially after toileting or diapering, and before any contact with food or surfaces involved in preparing and serving food.
2. Practice proper cleaning and sanitizing of surfaces. After surfaces are visibly clean, apply a sanitizer solution and leave it in contact with the surface for the time recommended on the product label.
3. Make an extra effort to practice frequent and correct hand washing, as well as cleaning and sanitizing of surfaces whenever an outbreak occurs.
4. Arrange for young children to receive the rotavirus vaccine.
5. Notify all parents when an outbreak occurs so they can watch for symptoms and make an extra effort to prevent the spread of the illness in their families.

Caregivers should

Notify parents.

Parents should

Follow caregiver's recommendations.

Child May Return to School or Child Care . . .

When the child is able to contain stool in the toilet for toilet-trained children, and for those still using diapers, when the child seems well and the stool consistency has not changed for a week.

Possible Problem: Shigella

What You Should Know

Shigella is an infection caused by the *Shigella* bacteria. It is transmitted via the fecal-oral route. Children under 5 years, adults who care for young children, and others living in crowded conditions are at increased risk. The incubation period is from 1 to 7 days. If left untreated, *Shigella* bacteria can live in the stool of an infected person for up to 4 weeks.

What You Should Look For

- Loose, watery stools with blood or mucus
- Fever
- Headache
- Convulsions
- Abdominal pain

What You Should Do

Caregivers and parents should

1. Practice proper hand washing, diapering, toileting and food-handling routines.
2. Do not allow children to share water play areas where water from a clean water source is not free flowing, such as water tables with one large bin into which all the children put their hands.

3. Notify the health department so that arrangements can be made to test the stool of everyone who has diarrhea.
4. Stop food handling or feeding of others by individuals with diarrhea.

Caregivers should

1. Notify parents.
2. Be sure everyone with diarrhea is tested.
3. Arrange for grouping together of children and adults who are well but still have positive stool tests for Shigella.

Parents should

1. Follow caregiver's recommendations.
2. Contact health care provider.

Child May Return to School or Child Care . . .

When treatment is complete and test results from stool cultures are negative.

Ear Pain

Possible Problem: Otitis Media (Middle Ear Infection)

What You Should Know

An infection of the middle ear most often occurs when mucus accumulates in the middle ear space. The mucus can come from a cold, allergy, or some other irritant of the respiratory tract. Mucus collects more easily in small children because the Eustachian tube that normally drains the middle ear is small, more horizontal, and easily blocked. Most middle ear infections are caused by viruses and resolve themselves in a day or two and are not contagious.

What You Should Look For

- Fever
- Pain or irritability
- Difficulty hearing
- Blocked ears
- Drainage
- Swelling around ear

What You Should Do

Caregivers and parents should

1. Keep the child with a respiratory infection well hydrated.
2. Prevent room air from becoming too dry. Dry air tends to dry out the secretions and make them thicker and harder to drain.
3. Ventilate indoor spaces with fresh outdoor air at least daily to reduce the concentration of germs in the air.
4. Follow the health provider's instructions to take care of the ear infection.
5. Do not allow children to drink from a bottle while lying on their backs. This position allows fluids to enter the Eustachian tube, causing irritation that can make it easier for an ear infection to start.
6. Watch for hearing loss or speech problems in children with recurring ear infections.

Caregivers should

Notify parents.

Parents should

1. Follow caregiver's recommendations.
2. Call child's health care provider for advice if the child has ear pain.

Child May Return to School or Child Care . . .

- Exclusion for ear infection is not necessary unless the child is too ill to participate or requires too much care to allow caregivers to meet the needs of the other children.
- Readmit when the child feels well enough to participate.

Eye Irritation/Pain

Possible Problem: Conjunctivitis (Pink Eye)

What You Should Know

Pink eye is an inflammation (i.e., redness, swelling) of the thin tissue covering the white part of the eye and the inside of the eyelids. There are several kinds of conjunctivitis, including bacterial, viral, allergic, and chemical. The infectious form is easily spread when a person touches discharge from an infected eye on surfaces and then touches his or her own eye area.

What You Should Look For

- Red, irritated, or painful eye(s)
- Yellow or watery drainage
- Eyelids temporarily stuck together from encrusted discharge when child awakens from sleep
- Watery drainage is most likely viral conjunctivitis, a sign of allergy or chemical irritation
- Pus or yellow drainage is most likely bacterial conjunctivitis; may be treated with an antibiotic

What You Should Do

Caregivers and parents should

1. Clean drainage from child's eye(s) with clean tissue or gauze pad and warm water, as needed. Wipe each eye outward from inner corner.
2. Discourage touching eye(s).
3. Wash hands thoroughly and encourage child to do the same.

Caregivers should

1. Have children with irritated eyes get advice from a health professional about what to do.
2. Contact the health department about how to keep infectious pink eye from spreading if more than one child has the infection.
3. Notify parents.

Parents should

1. Follow caregiver recommendations.
2. Call child's health care provider.
3. Apply antibiotic drops or ointment if prescribed.

Child May Return to School or Child Care . . .

Generally, children do not need to be excluded unless their eyes are red and they have green or yellow discharge (pus), which suggests the possibility of bacterial infection. If this is the problem, the child may return after the child starts treatment with an antibiotic and is able to participate without requiring more care than the staff can provide while they care for the other children in the group.

Possible Problem: Sty

What You Should Know

A sty is an infection of an oil gland inside the eyelid that creates a swelling, usually near the eyelashes.

What You Should Look For

- Appears as a lump in the eyelid, which may or may not be painful.

What You Should Do

Caregivers and parents should

1. Apply a warm wash cloth to the eye as often and for as long as possible during the day.
2. Encourage child not to touch his or her eyes.
3. Wash hands thoroughly and encourage child to do the same.

Caregivers should

Notify parents.

Parents should

1. Follow caregiver recommendations.
2. Call child's health care provider if no improvement.

Child May Return to School or Child Care . . .

No exclusion is necessary for a sty.

Fever

Possible Problem: Infection, Overheating, or Reaction to a Medication

What You Should Know

Fever alone is not harmful. When a child has an infection, raising the body temperature is part of the body's normal defenses. However, rapid elevation of body temperature sometimes can set off a febrile seizure in young children. This type of seizure is usually outgrown by 6 years of age. Fever is not a reason to send a child home. It is a reason to check for a cause of the fever and to monitor the child's behavior for other symptoms of illness.

What You Should Look For

- Flushed skin
- Tired
- Irritability
- Decreased activity
- 100°F axially (armpit)
- 101°F orally
- 102°F rectally
- Temperature taken with a tool that caregivers use in the child's ear or against the child's temple that gives a reading equal to oral or rectal temperature elevations

What You Should Do

Caregivers and parents should

1. Not give aspirin.
2. Check to see if the child is overheated, has had a medication or vaccine that might be causing the fever, and

whether the child is acting sick. If the child is overheated, cool the child off. If the child is acting sick, do what is needed for the child's behavior.

3. Get immediate medical advice for infants younger than 4 months of age with unexplained temperature elevations of 100°F axially (armpit) or 101°F rectally. Any infant younger than 2 months of age with these temperature elevations should get medical attention within an hour.

Caregivers should

Notify parents.

Parents should

1. Manage the problem that is causing the fever.
2. Give fever-reducing medication if instructed to do so by the child's health care provider.

Child May Return to School or Child Care . . .

Fever is not a reason to exclude a child from child care.

Headache

What You Should Know

Most headaches are minor and are caused by overexertion or stress. A headache might signal the beginning of illness. It also might signal a vision problem.

What You Should Look For

- Tired and irritable
- Holding head

What You Should Do

Caregivers and parents should

1. Have child rest in a quiet, darkened area.
2. Give any medication prescribed by the child's health care provider.
3. Notify health professional in case of sudden, severe headache with vomiting or a stiff neck that keeps the child from putting the chin down when asked to "look at your belly button." These symptoms might signal a life-threatening infection called meningitis.

Caregivers should

Report recurring headaches to parents.

Parents should

1. Have child rest in a quiet, darkened area.
2. Give medication if recommended by the child's health care provider.
3. Call child's health care provider for recurrent or severe headaches.

Child May Return to School or Child Care . . .

A headache is not a reason to exclude the child from care as long as the child can participate and does not require more care than the caregivers are able to provide.

Influenza

Possible Problem: Influenza Virus

What You Should Know

Influenza is a contagious disease caused by a group of respiratory viruses called the influenza viruses. It is spread through direct contact from sneezing and coughing. The contagious period lasts from the day before signs or symptoms appear until 7 days after the onset of flu.

What You Should Look For

- Sudden onset of fever
- Headache
- Chills
- Muscle aches and pains
- Sore throat
- Cough
- Mild pink eye
- Decreased energy
- Abdominal pain
- Nausea and vomiting

What You Should Do

Caregivers and parents should

1. Get vaccine for everyone involved in child care.
2. Practice careful and frequent hand washing after any contact with surfaces that might have nasal secretions on them.
3. Teach children to wash their hands after sneezing, coughing, or using a tissue.
4. Teach children to cover their noses and mouths with a shoulder or elbow, or use a tissue when sneezing or coughing. Dispose of facial tissues that contain nasal secretions after each use.
5. Avoid using any product that contains aspirin.

Caregivers should

1. Notify parents.
2. Work with the public health department to get everyone in the facility proper doses of influenza vaccine.

Parents should

1. Follow caregiver's recommendations.
2. Follow health care professional's recommendations.

Child May Return to School or Child Care . . .

- No exclusion from child care is necessary unless the child's behavior suggests that the child is too ill to participate and staff determine that they cannot care for the child without compromising their ability to care for the health and safety of the other children in the group.
- When symptoms resolve.

Itching Scalp

Possible Problem: *Pediculosis capitas* (Head Lice)

What You Should Know

Head lice is an infestation by a tiny parasitic insect on the scalp and hair. It is diagnosed by finding tiny yellow/white eggs, called nits, firmly attached to a shaft of hair; adult lice are harder to find. Nits can be found all along hair shafts and all over the head, but especially at the crown, the nape of the neck, and behind the ears.

Lice are transferred from person to person by crawling lice or through the sharing of personal items such as hats, combs, and brushes. It is not caused by uncleanliness. Lice cannot jump or fly and are not carried by cats or dogs.

All family members who have lice must be treated at the same time. Lice-killing shampoos are pesticides; therefore, use them according to the manufacturer's instructions. Combing out the hair with a special lice comb to remove nits and live lice is the most effective and safe approach, but it is very tedious. Household remedies do not work.

What You Should Look For

- Persistent itching on scalp
- Tiny red bites on scalp and on hairline
- Open sores and crusting

What You Should Do

Caregivers and parents should

1. Machine wash all washable items in hot water, followed by drying in the dryer, or send them to be dry cleaned. This includes bed linens, blankets, towels, clothing, jackets, and hats.
2. Use the high setting on the clothes dryer.
3. Place pillows and stuffed animals in dryer on hot setting for 30 minutes.
4. Place items that cannot be washed or dried in a closed plastic bag for 2 weeks.
5. Vacuum upholstered furniture, mattresses, rugs, car seats, and stuffed toys.
6. Do not use lice sprays.

Caregivers should

1. Notify the child's parents.
2. Notify all parents of a case of lice, but maintain confidentiality.

Parents should

1. Follow caregiver recommendations.
2. Treat with lice-killing shampoo as recommended by child's health care provider. Follow package directions and wear disposable gloves when applying shampoo.

3. Treat all family members who have lice at the same time.
4. Remove all nits and live lice with a small nit comb, available in most pharmacies, or with fingernails.
5. Check all family members' heads daily for 10 days.
6. Do not repeat treatment unless the product requires reapplication, and then do not do so again without consulting a health professional. Often, dandruff casts are mistaken for nits, or old empty nits (eggs) may be present but pose no problem.
7. Scrub hair brushes, combs, and hair accessories, and then soak them in very hot water for 10 minutes.

Child May Return to School or Child Care . . .

- The child does not have to be excluded before the end of the day.
- The child may return after treatment with lice-killing shampoo and thorough nit removal.

Lyme Disease

What You Should Know

Lyme disease is an infection caused by a type of bacteria known as *spirochetes* that is transmitted when particular types of ticks attach to a person's skin and feed on that person's blood. The common name for this type of tick is the deer tick. Lyme disease is not contagious and the incubation period is 3 to 31 days from the tick bite to appearance of a rash. It can be controlled by avoiding tick habitats and immediately removing any ticks from the body.

What You Should Look For

- Gradually expanding large, circular, or oval-shaped rash with a partial central clear area that appears after a tick bite
- Fever
- Headache
- Mild neck stiffness
- Flulike signs or symptoms
- Untreated Lyme disease may lead to arthritis, neurologic problems, cardiac problems, or meningitis

What You Should Do

Caregivers and parents should

1. Avoid tick habitats.
2. Apply permethrin to clothing or DEET to skin. You cannot use permethrin or DEET on infants under 2 months of age. Use DEET only between 10% and 30%. Lower concentrations are effective for shorter periods of time. DEET solutions of 10% are effective for about 2 hours.
3. Inspect children's skin and scalp after possible tick exposure.
4. Remove any ticks found on the child with tweezers (to grasp head).

Caregivers should

Notify parents.

Parents should

Consult child's health care provider if child develops a rash after a tick bite.

Child May Return to School or Child Care . . .

Child does not need to be excluded from care.

Measles

What You Should Know

Measles is a highly contagious and acute viral disease caused by the measles virus. Although there is a vaccine, outbreaks continue to occur among those who have not been protected by the vaccine. It is spread by direct contact with respiratory droplets (spread by sneezing or coughing). It is contagious from 1 to 2 days before the first signs or symptoms appear (usually 3 to 5 days before the rash) until 4 days after the appearance of the rash.

What You Should Look For

- Fever, cough, runny nose, and red, watery eyes
- Small red spots in mouth
- Appearance of rash at the hairline spreading downward over the body
- May have diarrhea or ear infection
- Complications may be serious and result in pneumonia, brain inflammation, convulsions, deafness, or mental retardation

What You Should Do

Caregivers and parents should

1. Make sure all adults and children have had two doses of MMR vaccine unless they were born before 1957. Review all immunization records for dates when each child, family member, and staff had the vaccine.
2. Practice proper hand washing.

3. Practice routine infection control measures.
4. Report the infection to the health department.

Caregivers should

1. Notify parents and follow instructions from the health department.
2. Exclude any children who might be exposed to the infection and who have either weakened immune systems or have not received the MMR vaccine for any reason. These children must be excluded for 2 weeks after the last child in the outbreak breaks out in the measles rash.

Parents should

1. Notify their health care professional.
2. Keep their child's vaccines up-to-date.

Child May Return to School or Child Care . . .

- Four days after the beginning of the rash.
- When the child is able to participate and staff determine that they can care for the child without compromising their ability to care for the health and safety of the other children in the group.

Mouth/Lip Sores

Possible Cause: Cold Sores (Herpes Simplex Virus)

What You Should Know

Herpes simplex virus is a viral disease that causes a variety of infections in different age groups. It is usually painful. Once someone is infected, the virus can become active again periodically. During the first infection, people shed the virus for at least a week and may continue to shed the virus for several weeks after signs or symptoms appear. People with recurrent infections shed the largest amount of virus for 3 to 4 days after signs or symptoms appear. The virus can be shed by people with no signs or symptoms of illness. This virus is spread by direct contact with the sore or by secretions from the sore that get on other surfaces, such as toys. Any adult or child who has mouth ulcers and blisters and does not have control of drooling or a sore on some other body area that cannot be completely covered should not be in a child care setting.

What You Should Look For

- Painful small fluid-filled blisters in mouth, on gums, or on lips
- Blisters that weep clear fluid and are slow to crust over
- Irritability
- Fever
- Tender, swollen lymph nodes

What You Should Do

Caregivers and parents should

1. Keep area of sores clean and dry.
2. Not touch an open cold sore.
3. Wash hands thoroughly whenever contact with infected material might have occurred, and also at routine times related to food handling, toileting, and contact with soiled surfaces.
4. Wash and sanitize mouthed toys, bottle nipples, and utensils that have come into contact with saliva or have been touched by children who are drooling and put fingers in their mouths.

Caregivers should

Notify parents, family members, and staff who may have been exposed so they can watch for symptoms.

Parents should

Follow caregiver recommendations.

Child May Return to School or Child Care . . .

- When an open sore has completely scabbed over or can be completely covered and when a child who has mouth sores and blisters is not drooling.
- The child is able to participate and staff determine that they can care for the child without compromising their ability to care for the health and safety of other children in the group.

Possible Cause: Hand, Foot, and Mouth Syndrome

What You Should Know

Hand, foot, and mouth syndrome is a common and usually mild viral infection that occurs more often in the summer and fall. The illness is more common among young children than older children or adults. It is transmitted from person to person through respiratory secretions and stool. The incubation period is 3 to 6 days. The illness commonly results in a fever and blisters in the child's mouth and on the palms and soles of the child's feet. The illness usually resolves on its own in about 1 week, but the virus can be present in stool for several weeks after infection starts. The virus can be shed by people who seem well.

What You Should Look For

- Tiny blisters or ulcers in the mouth and blisters on the fingers, palms of hands, and the soles of feet.
- May see common cold signs or symptoms with fever, sore throat, runny nose, and cough.

- The most troublesome finding often are the blisters in the mouth, which make it difficult for the child to eat or drink.
- Other signs or symptoms, such as vomiting and diarrhea, can occur.

What You Should Do

Caregivers and parents should

1. Report the infection to staff responsible for making decisions about care of ill children.
2. Encourage seeking of medical advice if the child seems very sick or uncomfortable.
3. Practice good hand-washing routines, especially after toileting or diaper changing.

Caregivers should

Encourage the child to drink small amounts often, to prevent dehydration.

Parents should

1. Consult a medical professional if the child seems very ill or very uncomfortable.
2. Not break blisters on hands and feet; they heal better if not broken.

Child May Return to School or Child Care . . .

- No exclusion from child care is necessary unless the child is unable to participate and staff determine that they cannot care for the child without compromising their ability to care for the health and safety of the other children in the group.
- Note: Exclusion will not reduce disease transmission, because some children may shed the virus without becoming recognizably ill and the virus may be shed for weeks in the stool after the child seems well.

Possible Cause: Thrush

What You Should Know

Thrush is a yeast infection in the mouth that seldom occurs in infants over 6 months of age. The fungus is widespread in the environment, especially in warm and moist tissues. The fungus causes disease when it overgrows healthy germs in the lining of the mouth. This infection is usually treated with antifungal medication.

What You Should Look For

White patches on the inside of cheeks and on gums and tongue.

What You Should Do

Caregivers and parents should

1. Wash hands thoroughly.
2. Carefully wash and sanitize all items that might reinfect child, such as nipples, pacifiers, and mouthed toys.
3. Do not allow babies to share mouthed toys, pacifiers, or bottles that have not been washed and sanitized.
4. Follow the instructions of the child's health care provider for medication and treatment to reduce the amount of yeast to levels that do not cause illness.

Caregivers should

Notify parents.

Parents should

Follow health care professional's and caregiver's recommendations.

Child May Return to School or Child Care . . .

Children with thrush do not need to be excluded from the group setting.

Skin Eruptions and Rashes

Possible Cause: Chicken Pox

What You Should Know

Chicken pox is a highly contagious, common viral illness lasting approximately 1 week. The incubation period is about 14 to 16 days, occasionally as short as 10 days and as long as 21 days after contact. It is most contagious from 1 to 2 days before the rash appears until all the blisters have scabs and no new blisters are forming. Shared air or contact with body fluids from an infected person spreads the virus. A vaccine is recommended for everyone who has not already had chicken pox. Shingles is the recurrent form of the chicken pox virus in someone in whom the virus remains alive; it can cause illness from time to time throughout life.

What You Should Look For

- Rash of red bumps appears primarily on face and trunk as fluid-filled bubbles that break, weep, and scab.
- Rash can also appear on arms, legs, or any mucous membrane surface, such as inside the mouth, throat, eyes, and vagina.
- Fever
- Runny nose
- Cough
- Itching

What You Should Do

Caregivers and parents should

1. Avoid products that contain aspirin or aspirin-like chemicals (salicylates).
2. Follow the advice of the child's health care professional for management of symptoms, such as use of acetaminophen for fever and cool baths to control itching and prevent secondary infection from scratching.
3. Watch for chicken pox to develop in other family members or playmates for 3 weeks.

Caregivers should

1. Notify parents.
2. Notify health authorities when a case occurs in group care so outbreak measures can be started.
3. Check the immunization records of all people over 12 months of age who are involved in any way with the child-care program to be sure each person is immunized.
4. Be sure that anyone who has shingles (adult recurrence of the chicken pox virus) covers their blisters so that the virus shed from these sores does not spread to others.

Parents should

1. Encourage child to drink clear fluids.
2. Bathe child in cool water to relieve itching.
3. Some children may be more comfortable if their itchy spots are painted with a thin film of calamine lotion. Letting a child paint her own itchy spots may be particularly comforting.
4. Trim child's fingernails or put mittens on infant to prevent scratching, which can infect open lesions and lead to scarring.

5. Consult the child's health care provider if the child seems very uncomfortable or ill.
6. Be sure all family members who have not already had chicken pox and who are older than 12 months of age receive the vaccine as quickly as possible.

Child May Return to School or Child Care . . .

When all blisters have crusted, approximately 7 days.

Possible Cause: Fifth Disease

What You Should Know

Fifth disease is a mild viral illness, harmless for most children. The rash usually comes 1 to 3 weeks after the infection. The incubation period is 4 to 14 days, but may last up to 21 days. It is contagious until the appearance of the rash. It spreads through contact with throat and mouth secretions or exposure to blood that contains the virus. It can be serious for an unborn child (a fetus) or for children with some chronic illnesses, such as sickle cell anemia and thalessemia, or with suppressed immune systems, such as leukemia and AIDS patients. One bout of infection is believed to provide lifelong immunity. About half of all adults have already had the disease, and 90% have had it by the time they reach old age.

What You Should Look For

- Fever
- Muscle aches
- Joint pain
- Headache
- Red "slapped-cheek" rash
- Lacelike rash

What You Should Do

Caregivers and parents should

1. Care for symptoms of illness according to the recommendations of the child's health care provider.
2. Notify all staff and parents because of possible health risks to unborn babies and to children with serious illnesses.
3. A pregnant woman who is exposed to fifth disease should consult her health care provider for the possibility of having a blood test to determine whether her baby is at risk.

Caregivers should

Notify parents and staff that fifth disease is common in childhood and that hand washing is the best protection from infection.

Parents should

Contact child's health care provider if the child has a chronic illness that makes the child especially vulnerable to infection.

Child May Return to School or Child Care . . .

- Child need not be excluded from school or child care unless the child has sickle cell disease or a compromised immune system. Children with these conditions may shed large amounts of virus and become very ill.
- No exclusion is necessary if the child is able to participate and the staff determine that they can care for the child without compromising their ability to care for the health and safety of the other children in the group.

Possible Cause: Heat Rash (Prickly Heat)

What You Should Know

Prickly heat is experienced mostly by infants and young children. It occurs during hot and humid weather, when production of a lot of sweat swells the tissues around the opening of the sweat glands, blocking the openings of the tubes that carry the sweat to the surface. This makes little red bumps around the sweat duct openings.

What You Should Look For

- Tiny red bumps in areas that tend to be moist
- Commonly seen in skin folds of neck and on upper chest, arms, legs, and diaper area

What You Should Do

Caregivers and parents should

1. Pay special attention to skin folds that stay wet with perspiration, urine, or drool.
2. Use cool water to remove body oil and sweat, and then dry the area.
3. Leave areas open to air, without clothing.
4. Use air conditioning or a fan blowing gently on child to keep the child cool.
5. Do not apply skin ointments.

Caregivers should

Notify parents.

Parents should

1. Follow caregiver recommendations.
2. Dress the child in clothing that keeps the skin cool and dry.

Child May Return to School or Child Care . . .

Child need not be excluded from school or child care.

Possible Cause: Impetigo

What You Should Know

Impetigo is a *streptococcal* or *staphylococcal* bacterial skin infection that can develop after an insect bite, cut, or other break in the skin. It can develop in any skin injury such as an insect bite, a cut, or irritation caused by a runny nose. Children can spread the infection to other parts of the body by scratching. They can also spread the germs to others in close contact by direct touching or touching a surface that another child touches. Impetigo can occur anytime, but is most common in warm weather when cuts and scrapes from outdoor play are likely to occur.

What You Should Look For

Red pimples or fluid-filled blisters or an oozing rash covered by crusted yellow scabs.

What You Should Do

Caregivers and parents should

1. Discourage scratching.
2. Trim fingernails.
3. Do not permit sharing of towels or face cloths.
4. Wash hands thoroughly.
5. Cover sores until they are healed.
6. Observe rash and note any improvement or worsening.

Caregivers should

1. Notify parents to watch for sores.
2. If the child cannot be picked up promptly, wash the affected area with soap and water and then cover any exposed sores until the parents can arrange to remove the child for treatment.
3. In the event that more than one child in a group has been infected, contact the health department about control measures. The problem could involve antibiotic-resistant *staphylococcal* bacteria.

Parents should

1. Follow caregiver recommendations.
2. Call child's health care provider for a treatment plan.
3. Clean infected area with soap and water and try to gently remove crusty scabs.
4. Cover infected area loosely to allow airflow for healing and to prevent contact that would spread the infection to others or to other parts of the child's body.

Child May Return to School or Child Care . . .

- 24 hours after treatment is started with an antibiotic ointment or oral antibiotic medication.
- When the child is able to participate and staff determine that they can care for the child without compromising their ability to care for the health and safety of the other children in the group.

Possible Cause: Ringworm

What You Should Know

Ringworm is a fungal infection that can affect the body, feet, or scalp. It is mildly contagious. On the skin of the body or limbs, the infection causes round or oval, red, scaly patches with raised edges and a clear area in the center. The fungus may grow between the toes causing cracking and peeling. On the scalp, the fungus causes patchy areas of dandruff-like scaling with or without hair loss. Ringworm spreads from person to person by direct contact; by sharing combs, brushes, hats, hair ornaments, towels, clothing, or bedding; or by contact with infected people or surfaces contaminated by people who have a ringworm lesion. Skin infections are treated with an antifungal topical cream. Scalp infections require an oral medication that must be taken for weeks. It is no longer contagious once treatment is started.

What You Should Look For

- Red, circular patches with raised edges and a clear area in the center
- Cracking and peeling of skin between toes
- Patchy areas of dandruff-like scaling with or without hair loss
- Redness and scaling of scalp with broken hairs or patches of hair loss

What You Should Do

Caregivers and parents should

1. Alert exposed staff and families to watch for symptoms.
2. Wash hands thoroughly and encourage child to do the same.
3. Make sure the child takes prescribed medication for the recommended time for the treatment to be effective.

4. Avoid sharing of dress-up articles or other clothing unless the fabric is washed between users or disposed of after one person uses it.

Caregivers should

1. Notify parents to remove the child at the end of the program day and not return until treatment is started.
2. On arrival and by observation while children are in care, note any areas of skin or scalp that might be affected.
3. Restructure dress-up play areas or any place where clothing or headgear is shared to ensure that the equipment is laundered or sanitized between uses by different children.

Parents should

Follow the health care professional's recommended treatment plan.

Child May Return to School or Child Care . . .

Once treatment is started.

Possible Cause: Roseola

What You Should Know

Roseola is a viral illness occurring in young children between 6 and 24 months of age. The incubation period is 9 to 10 days. It is mildly contagious. One bout provides immunity.

What You Should Look For

- A persistent high fever (103°F or higher) for 3 to 7 days
- Fever may cause seizure activity
- Often the child is not very ill when the fever is present
- Red, raised rash lasting from hours to several days that becomes apparent the day the fever breaks—usually the fourth day

What You Should Do

Caregivers and parents should

1. Notify exposed family members and staff to watch for symptoms.
2. Inform and reassure parents about the nature of the illness and that once the rash appears, the child is on the way to being well.

Caregivers should

Notify parents.

Parents should

Follow the advice of the child's health care provider about managing the fever.

Child May Return to School or Child Care . . .

The child does not need to be excluded if the child's fever is not accompanied by a behavior change and if the child is able to participate and if staff determine that they can care for the child without compromising their ability to care for the health and safety of the other children in the group.

Possible Cause: Scabies

What You Should Know

Scabies is a parasitic infestation caused by mites that burrow under the superficial layer of skin. The incubation period is 4 to 6 weeks for people who have never had the condition before, and 1 to 4 days for those who have been infested previously. The feces of the mites that are left under the skin cause intense itching. It may be diagnosed by the appearance of the rash or by a skin scraping in which the mite or egg is seen. The mites are transferred by person-to-person contact and by the sharing of bedding, towels, or clothing. The child and all family members must be treated at home at the same time with prescription mite-killing cream or lotion. Itching might last 2 to 4 weeks after treatment. Scabies affects people from all socioeconomic levels without regard to age or personal hygiene.

What You Should Look For

- Rash, severe itching (increased at night)
- Itchy red bumps or blisters found on skin folds between the fingers, toes, wrists, elbows, armpits, waistline, thighs, penis, abdomen, and lower buttocks
- Children younger than 2 years are likely to be infested on the head, neck, palms, and soles of feet or in a diffuse distribution over the body

What You Should Do

Caregivers and parents should

1. Machine wash all washable items in hot water, including bed linens, blankets, towels, clothing, jackets, and hats.
2. Use the high setting on the clothes dryer.
3. Place pillows and stuffed animals in a dryer on hot setting for 30 minutes.
4. Leave items that cannot be washed or dried in a closed plastic bag for at least 4 days.
5. Discourage child from scratching.

Caregivers should

1. Notify the family of the child with symptoms.
2. Notify exposed family members and staff to watch for symptoms.

Parents should

1. Follow caregiver recommendations.
2. Follow package directions when applying the mite-killing lotion.
3. Treat all infected family members at the same time.

Child May Return to School or Child Care . . .

After treatment is completed (treatment usually requires application of a lotion that stays on the skin overnight and then is washed off).

Possible Cause: Scarlet Fever (Scarlatina)

What You Should Know

Scarlatina is a streptococcal bacterial infection that causes a generalized illness with a rash. It is the same type of bacteria that causes strep throat and is not more serious than strep throat. The incubation period is 2 to 5 days. It is contagious and spreads from person to person by direct contact or by inhaling tiny droplets of infected secretions from the nose. Many people carry the strep bacteria in their nose and throat and are not ill. When the strep bacteria takes over as the most common germ in the tissue and causes illness, it must be treated with an antibiotic.

What You Should Look For

- Rash appears primarily on trunk and is most intense at underarms, on groin, behind the knees, and on the inner thighs.
- Rash is slightly raised fine bumps that make the skin feel like fine sandpaper.
- Painful sore throat in children over 3 years of age; persistent nasal discharge and foul odor from the mouth in children under 3 years of age.

- High fever
- Tongue has white coating that changes to the appearance of a strawberry after 4 to 5 days.
- Nausea, vomiting, and decreased appetite
- Swollen lymph nodes in the neck (swollen glands)
- Headache
- Skin peels after 1 week

What You Should Do

Caregivers and parents should

1. Have a diagnosis made by a health care professional.
2. Follow the instructions of the health care professional for treatment.
3. Encourage child to drink clear fluids.
4. Wash hands thoroughly after caring for child to reduce chance of spreading infection to yourself and others.

Caregivers should

Notify parents of the child and the families who may have been exposed to the infection.

Parents should

1. Wash hands thoroughly after caring for child.
2. Call child's health care provider to arrange for a diagnosis and treatment.

Child May Return to School or Child Care . . .

- 24 hours after antibiotic treatment has started.
- When the child is able to participate and if staff determine that they can care for the child without compromising their ability to care for the health and safety of the other children in the group.

Sore Throat

Possible Cause: Viral Sore Throat

What You Should Know

A viral sore throat is the most common cause of a sore throat. It is contagious, but it will get better without treatment. More than 90% of sore throats are viral.

What You Should Look For

A throat that feels raw.

What You Should Do

Caregivers and parents should

1. Encourage the child to drink fluids.
2. Wash hands thoroughly after caring for child.
3. Do not allow child to share mouthed toys, pacifiers, bottles, cups, or eating utensils.

Caregivers should

1. Notify parents about the child's illness.
2. If two or more children in the same group have the same symptoms, notify the families of the exposed children to watch for similar symptoms.

Parents should

1. Follow caregiver recommendations.
2. Call child's health care provider for throat culture if symptoms persist for more than 2 days.

Child May Return to School or Child Care . . .

Do not exclude unless the child cannot swallow, is drooling excessively, having breathing difficulty, has fever with a behavior change, or the child is unable to participate or if staff determine that they cannot care for the child without compromising their ability to care for the health and safety of the other children in the group.

Possible Cause: "Strep" Throat

What You Should Know

A strep throat is a *streptococcal* bacterial infection. It occurs much less often than a viral throat infection, but it requires treatment. The incubation period is 2 to 5 days. It is contagious and spreads from person to person by direct contact or by inhaling tiny droplets of infected secretions from the nose. Many people carry the strep bacteria in their nose and throat and are not ill. When the strep bacteria takes over as the most common germ in the tissue and causes illness, it must be treated with an antibiotic. A laboratory test is required to diagnose it with certainty.

What You Should Look For

Some of the following symptoms may be present:

- Sore throat
- Fever
- Stomachache
- Headache
- Swollen lymph nodes in neck
- Decreased appetite

Strep throat is much less likely if there is:

- Runny nose
- Cough
- Congestion

Children younger than 3 years rarely have a sore throat. Most commonly, these children have a persistent nasal discharge (which may be associated with a foul odor from the mouth), fever, irritability, and loss of appetite.

What You Should Do

Caregivers and parents should

1. Wash hands thoroughly after caring for child.
2. Do not allow child to share mouthed toys, pacifiers, bottles, cups, or eating utensils.

Caregivers should

Notify parents of the child and the families who may have been exposed to the infection.

Parents should

1. Contact the child's health care provider to obtain a diagnosis and treatment plan.
2. Complete entire course of antibiotic treatment to prevent relapse, even if child appears to recover quickly.

Child May Return to School or Child Care . . .

- 24 hours after antibiotic treatment has started.
- When the child is able to participate and if staff determine that they can care for the child without compromising their ability to care for the health and safety of the other children in the group.

Tooth Pain

Possible Cause: Bottlemouth Syndrome

What You Should Know

Bottlemouth syndrome is a special form of tooth decay in very young children. It is caused by prolonged exposure to milk or other liquids containing sugar at naptime and bedtime and by carrying sugary beverages or milk around during the day. It is most common in upper front teeth. Treatment often requires oral surgery with general anesthesia.

What You Should Look For

- Red gums
- Irritated mouth
- Teeth that do not look normal

What You Should Do

Caregivers and parents should

1. Not give child a bottle of milk or juice (or any fluid containing sugar) at naptime, bedtime, or to carry around during the day. Confine feedings to specific meal and snack times.
2. Give the child water after a feeding to rinse the sugary liquid off the teeth.
3. Give only water, or eliminate the sleep-time bottle.

Caregivers should

Notify parents about the need to have the child's teeth examined by a health care professional.

Parents should

Follow caregiver recommendations.

Child May Return to School or Child Care . . .

Child need not be excluded from school or child care.

Possible Cause: Cavities

What You Should Know

Cavities are caused by sticky foods that leave sugar coating on teeth. This sugar feeds the bacteria in the mouth that then produce acid that destroys the hard surface of the teeth. Some of the bacteria that do the most damage are transferred from the mouth of caregivers to the children.

What You Should Look For

- Irritated mouth
- Sore gums
- Abnormal appearance or color of the teeth or discolorations on the teeth

What You Should Do

Caregivers and parents should

1. Avoid giving child sticky foods between meals that cling to teeth and cause decay, such as gummy fruit-flavored treats, caramel candy, and licorice.
2. Encourage child to eat pretzels, raw vegetables, fresh fruit, and yogurt as snack foods.

3. Encourage child to brush or rinse teeth after snacks and meals.
4. Follow the child's oral health care provider's recommendations about the use of fluoride, which may include application of varnishes and the use of rinses, fluoride supplements, or special toothpastes.

Caregivers should

Notify parents.

Parents should

Follow caregiver and child's oral health professional's recommendations.

Child May Return to School or Child Care . . .

Child need not be excluded from school or child care.

Possible Cause: Teething

What You Should Know

Teething is gum pain caused by newly erupting teeth. It can cause exaggerated crankiness. It can be very painful and cause sleepless nights. It does not cause fever, but it can lead to the child getting an infection by putting objects in the mouth.

What You Should Look For

- Crankiness
- Sleepless nights

What You Should Do

Caregivers and parents should

1. Provide teething toys for the child to chew.
2. Consult the child's health care professional about using pain-reducing medications, especially when the child is trying to sleep.

Caregivers should

Notify parents.

Parents should

Follow caregiver recommendations.

Child May Return to School or Child Care . . .

Child need not be excluded from school or child care if the child is able to participate and if staff determine that they can care for the child without compromising their ability to care for the health and safety of the other children in the group.

Upper Respiratory Infection

Possible Cause: Common Cold

What You Should Know

An upper respiratory infection is a viral infection of the upper respiratory tract (nose, throat, ears, and eyes). It can also result from a bacterial infection called *Mycoplasma*. The incubation period is between 2 to 14 days, and the child is contagious a few days before signs or symptoms appear and while clear runny secretions are present. It is spread by direct or close contact with mouth and nose secretions or through touching contaminated objects.

What You Should Look For

- Cough
- Sore or scratchy throat or tonsillitis
- Runny nose
- Sneezing or nasal discharge
- Watery eyes
- Fever is low grade or does not exist.
- Earache that may come after the secretions from a cold thicken and block up the drainage tube that goes from inside the ear into the throat.

What You Should Do

Caregivers and parents should

- Practice good hand-washing techniques.
- Teach children to "give coughs and sneezes a cold shoulder" by using their shoulder or elbow to cover their noses and mouths when they cough or sneeze and do not have a facial tissue handy.
- Teach children to wash their hands after sneezing, coughing, or handling tissues.
- Dispose of facial tissues immediately.
- Sanitize surfaces that are touched frequently (toys, doorknobs, tables).
- Ventilate rooms with fresh outdoor air.

Caregivers should

Notify parents about practices to reduce the transmission of cold viruses.

Parents should

Follow caregiver's recommendations.

Child May Return to School or Child Care . . .

Child does not need to be excluded unless the child is unable to participate or if staff determine that they cannot care for the child without compromising their ability to care for the health and safety of the other children in the group.

Urination, Painful

Possible Cause: Urinary Tract Infection

What You Should Know

Most urinary tract infections are caused by bacteria. Urinary tract infections are more common in girls than boys because girls have a shorter tube that connects the bladder to the outside (the urethra). Also, in girls, this tube is close to the anus, and bacteria in stool can easily get into the opening to the urinary tract. Boys do not usually get urinary tract infections unless they have some other health problem. Among boys with a condition that predisposes them to urinary tract infection, those who are uncircumcised are more likely to develop a urinary tract infection.

What You Should Look For

- Pain when urinating
- Increased frequency of urinating
- Fever
- Loss of potty training

What You Should Do

Caregivers and parents should

1. Encourage children to drink enough fluids to keep their urine light yellow or clear like water. Very young children can learn that a dark urine color means they need to drink more.

2. Teach girls to wipe only from front to back after toileting.

Caregivers should

Notify child's parents about any symptoms of urinary infection and ask that the family consult the child's health care provider.

Parents should

1. Follow caregiver recommendations.

2. Call child's health care provider promptly.

3. Have child give urine specimen for testing and be treated as appropriate to the condition that the health care professional diagnoses.

4. Avoid using bubble baths; these products are common causes of irritation of urinary and genital tissues that makes it easier for a urinary infection to start, especially in girls.

Child May Return to School or Child Care . . .

Child need not be excluded from school or child care if the child is able to participate and if staff determine that they can care for the child without compromising their ability to care for the health and safety of the other children in the group.

Vomiting

Possible Cause: Viral Gastrointestinal Infection

What You Should Know

Viral gastrointestinal infections often are contagious. They are less often caused by food poisoning or emotional upset.

What You Should Look For

- Diarrhea
- Vomiting
- Cramps

What You Should Do

Caregivers and parents should

1. Remove child from the group if vomiting occurs more than once.
2. Give no food or fluid until 1 hour after vomiting has stopped.
3. Give fluids in small enough amounts so that no vomiting occurs, starting with an ounce, then in 15 minutes, give half as much if that amount produces vomiting or twice as much in the next 15 minutes if that amount stays down.

Caregivers should

Notify parents.

Parents should

1. Manage vomiting.
2. Consult the child's health care professional as soon as possible if:

- The vomiting continues, and the child has not urinated in 8 hours.
- The vomiting is associated with persistent abdominal pain.
- The vomit appears green or bloody.
- The child has had a recent head injury.
- The child looks or acts very ill.

Child May Return to School or Child Care . . .

When the child is able to participate and if staff determine that they can care for the child without compromising their ability to care for the health and safety of the other children in the group.

CHOKING/CPR

LEARN AND PRACTICE CPR (CARDIOPULMONARY RESUSCITATION)

IF ALONE WITH A CHILD WHO IS CHOKING...

1. SHOUT FOR HELP. 2. START RESCUE EFFORTS. 3. CALL 911 OR YOUR LOCAL EMERGENCY NUMBER.

YOU SHOULD START FIRST AID FOR CHOKING IF...	*DO NOT* START FIRST AID FOR CHOKING IF...
• The child cannot breathe at all (the chest is not moving up and down). • The child cannot cough or talk, or looks blue. • The child is found unconscious. (Go to CPR.)	• The child can breathe, cry, or talk. • The child can cough, sputter, or move air at all. The child's normal reflexes are working to clear the airway.

FOR INFANTS YOUNGER THAN 1 YEAR

INFANT CHOKING

If the infant is choking and is unable to breathe, cough, cry, or speak, follow these steps. Have someone call 911, or if you are alone call 911 as soon as possible.

1 GIVE FIVE BACK SLAPS

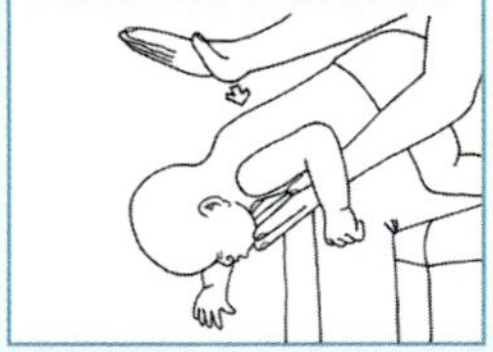

ALTERNATING WITH

2 GIVE FIVE CHEST THRUSTS

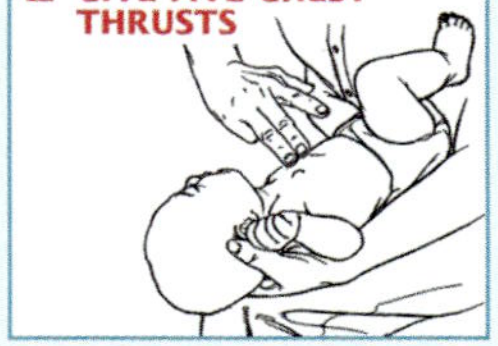

Alternate back slaps and chest thrusts until the object is dislodged or the infant becomes unconscious. If the infant becomes unconscious, begin CPR.

INFANT CPR

To be used when the infant is unconscious or when breathing stops.

1 OPEN AIRWAY

- Open airway (tilt head, lift chin).
- Take 5 to 10 seconds to check if the child is breathing after the airway is opened. **Look** for up and down movement of the chest and abdomen. **Listen** for breath sounds at the nose and mouth. **Feel** for breath on your cheek. If opening the airway results in breathing, other than an occasional gasp, do not give breaths.
- If there is no breathing **look** for a foreign object in the mouth. **If you can see** an object in the infant's mouth, sweep it out carefully with your finger. Then attempt rescue breathing. **Do NOT** try a blind finger sweep if the object is not seen, because it could be pushed farther into the throat.

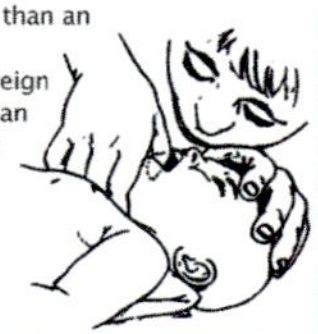

2 RESCUE BREATHING

- **Position** head and chin with both hands as shown head gently tilted back, chin lifted.
- Take a normal breath (not a deep breath).
- **Seal** your mouth over the infant's mouth and nose.
- Give 2 breaths, each rescue breath over 1 second with a pause between breaths. Each breath should make the chest rise.

If no rise or fall after the first breath, repeat steps 1 and 2. If still no rise or fall, continue with step 3 (below).

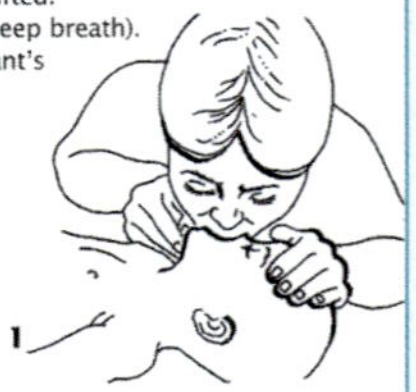

3 CHEST COMPRESSIONS

- Place 2 fingers of 1 hand on the breastbone just below the nipple line.
- Compress chest ⅓ to ½ the depth of the chest.
- Alternate 30 compressions with 2 breaths.
- Compress chest at rate of 100 times per minute.

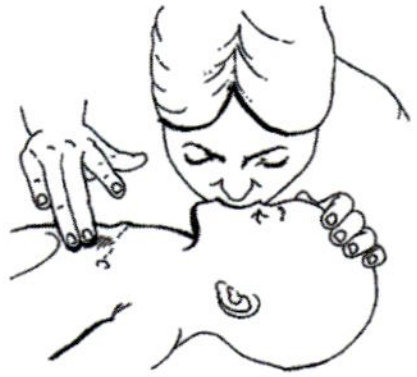

Be sure someone calls 911 as soon as possible. If you are alone, call 911 or your local emergency number after 5 cycles of breaths and chest compressions (about 2 minutes).

FOR CHILDREN 1 TO 8 YEARS OF AGE*

CHILD CHOKING

If the child is choking and is unable to breathe, cough, cry, or speak, follow these steps. Have someone call 911, or if you are alone call 911 as soon as possible.

CONSCIOUS

FIVE ABDOMINAL THRUSTS just above the navel and well below the bottom tip of the breastbone and rib cage. Give each thrust with enough force to produce an artificial cough designed to relieve airway obstruction.

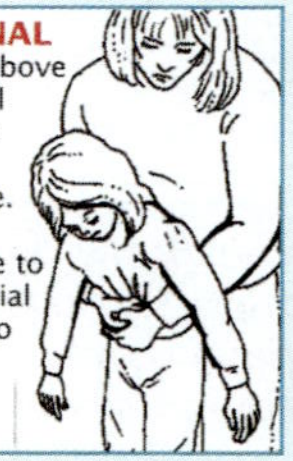

If the child becomes unconscious, begin CPR.

The information contained in this publication should not be used as a substitute for the medical advice of your pediatrician. There may be variations in treatment that your pediatrician may recommend based on the individual facts and circumstances.

CHILD CPR

To be used when the child is **UNCONSCIOUS** or when breathing stops.

1 OPEN AIRWAY

- Open airway (tilt head, lift chin).
- Take 5 to 10 seconds to check if the child is breathing after the airway is opened. **Look** for up and down movement of the chest and abdomen. **Listen** for breath sounds at the nose and mouth. **Feel** for breath on your cheek. If opening the airway results in breathing, other than an occasional gasp, do not give breaths.
- If there is no breathing **look** for a foreign object in the mouth. **If you can see** an object in the child's mouth, sweep it out carefully with your finger. Then attempt rescue breathing. **Do NOT** try a blind finger sweep if the object is not seen, because it could be pushed farther into the throat.

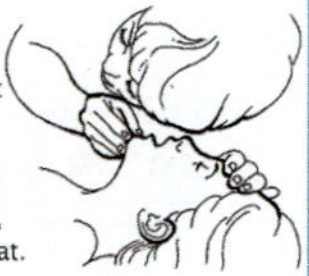

2 RESCUE BREATHING

- **Position** head and chin with both hands as shown head gently tilted back, chin lifted.
- Take a normal breath (not a deep breath).
- **Seal** your mouth over the child's mouth.
- **Pinch** the child's nose.
- Give 2 breaths, each rescue breath over 1 second with a pause between breaths. Each breath should make the chest rise and fall.

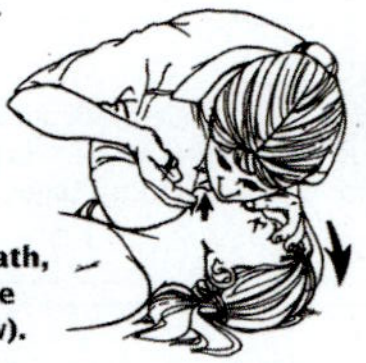

If no rise or fall after the first breath, repeat steps 1 and 2. If still no rise or fall, continue with step 3 (below).

3 CHEST COMPRESSIONS

Place heel of 1 hand over the lower half of the breastbone OR use 2 hands: place heel of 1 hand over the lower half of the breastbone, then place other hand over first hand and intertwine fingers (to keep them off of the chest).

- Compress chest ⅓ to ½ depth of chest.
- Alternate 30 compressions with 2 breaths.
- Compress chest at rate of 100 times per minute.

Check for signs of normal breathing, coughing, or movement after every 5 cycles (about 2 minutes).

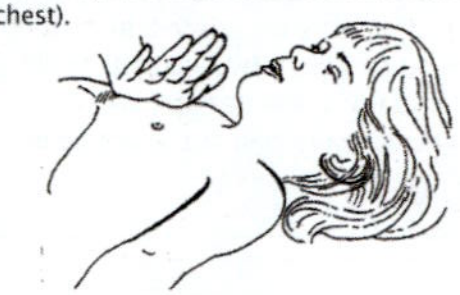

1-hand technique

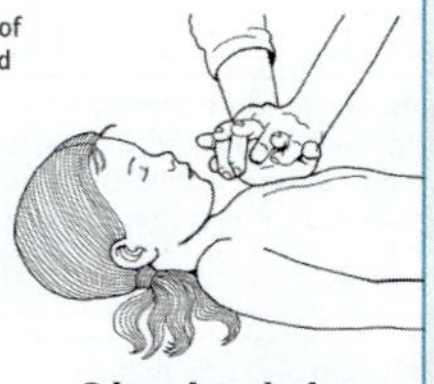

2-hand technique

Be sure someone calls 911 as soon as possible. If you are alone, call 911 or your local emergency number after 5 cycles of breaths and chest compressions (about 2 minutes).

***For children 8 years and older, adult recommendations for choking/CPR apply.**

If at any time an object is coughed up or the infant/child starts to breathe, call 911 or your local emergency number.

Ask your pediatrician for information on choking/CPR instructions for children older than 8 years and for information on an approved first aid or CPR course in your community.

Turn Over for First Aid Instructions

HE0418, Updated 4/06

FIRST AID

Call 911 or an emergency number for a severely ill or injured child. Call 1-800-222-1222 (Poison Center) if you have a poison emergency.

Poisons

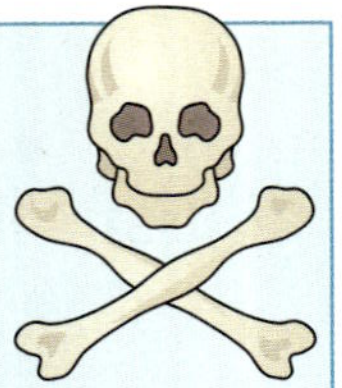

If the child has been exposed to or ingested a poison, call the Poison Center at 1-800-222-1222. A poison expert in your area is available 24 hours a day, 7 days a week.

Swallowed Poisons Any nonfood substance is a potential poison. Do not give anything by mouth or induce vomiting. Call the Poison Center right away. Do not delay, but try to have the substance label or name available when you call.

Fumes, Gases, or Smoke Get the child into fresh air and call 911 or the fire department. If the child is not breathing, start CPR and continue until help arrives. (Please see next page.)

Skin Exposure If acids, lye, pesticides, chemicals, poisonous plants, or any potentially poisonous substance comes in contact with a child's skin, eyes, or hair, brush off any residual material while wearing rubber gloves, if possible. Remove contaminated clothing. Wash skin, eyes, or hair with large amount of water or mild soap and water. Do not scrub. Call the Poison Center for further advice.

If a child is unconscious, becoming drowsy, having convulsions, or having trouble breathing, call 911 or an emergency number. Bring the poisonous substance (safely contained) with you to the hospital.

Fever

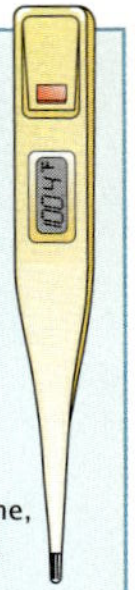

Fever in children is usually caused by infection. It also can be caused by chemicals, poisons, medicines, an environment that is too hot, or an extreme level of overactivity. Take the child's temperature to see if he has a fever. Most pediatricians consider any thermometer reading above 100.4°F (38°C) a sign of a fever. However, the way the child looks and acts is more important than how high the child's temperature is. Call the pediatrician right away if the child has a fever and:

- Appears very ill, is unusually drowsy, or is very fussy
- Has other symptoms such as a stiff neck, severe headache, severe sore throat, severe ear pain, an unexplained rash, or repeated vomiting or diarrhea
- Has a condition causing immune suppression (such as sickle cell disease, cancer, or the taking of steroids)
- Has had a first seizure
- Is younger than 2 months and has a temperature of 100.4°F (38°C) or higher
- Has been in a very hot place, such as an overheated car

To make the child more comfortable, dress him in light clothing, give him cool liquids to drink, and keep him calm. The pediatrician may recommend fever medicines. Do not use aspirin to treat a child's fever. Aspirin has been linked with Reye syndrome, a serious disease that affects the liver and brain.

Eye Injuries

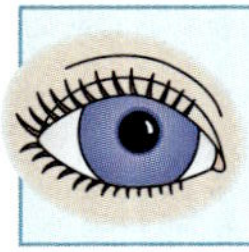

If anything is splashed in the eye, flush gently with water for at least 15 minutes. Call the Poison Center or the pediatrician for further advice. Any injured or painful eye should be seen by a doctor. Do **NOT** touch or rub an injured eye. Do **NOT** apply medicine. Do **NOT** remove objects stuck in the eye. Cover the painful or injured eye with a paper cup or eye shield until you can get medical help. The child may need a tetanus booster.

Fainting

Check the child's airway and breathing. If necessary, call 911 and begin rescue breathing and CPR. (Please see next page). If vomiting has occurred, turn the child onto one side to prevent choking. Elevate the feet above the level of the heart (about 12 inches). Do **NOT** give the child anything to drink.

Nosebleeds

Keep the child in a sitting position with the head tilted slightly forward. Apply firm, steady pressure to both nostrils by squeezing them between your thumb and index finger for 10 minutes. If bleeding continues, or is very heavy, call the pediatrician or seek emergency care

General

- Know how to get help.
- Make sure the area is safe for you and the child.
- When possible, personal protective equipment (gloves, etc) should be used.
- Position the child appropriately if her airway needs to be opened or CPR (cardiopulmonary resuscitation) is needed. (Please see other side.)
- DO NOT MOVE A CHILD WHO MAY HAVE A NECK OR BACK INJURY (from a fall, motor vehicle crash, or other injury, or if they say their neck or back hurts).
- Look for anything (medical jewelry, paperwork, etc) that may give you information about health problems

Fractures and Sprains

If an injured area is painful, swollen, or deformed, or if motion causes pain, wrap it in a towel or soft cloth and make a splint with cardboard or other firm material to hold the arm or leg in place. Apply ice or a cold compress wrapped in thin cloth for not more than 20 minutes. Call the pediatrician or seek emergency care. If there is a break in the skin near the fracture or if you can see the bone, cover the area with a clean bandage, make a splint as described above, and seek emergency care.

If the foot or hand below the injured part is cold or discolored (blue or pale), seek emergency care right away.

Convulsions, Seizures

If the child is breathing, lay her on her side to prevent choking. Make sure the child is safe from objects that could injure her. Be sure to protect her head. Do not put anything in the child's mouth. Loosen any tight clothing. Start rescue breathing if the child is blue or not breathing. (Please see next page). Call 911 or an emergency number for a prolonged seizure (more than 5 minutes).

Teeth

Baby Teeth If knocked out or broken, apply clean gauze to control bleeding and call the pediatric dentist.

Permanent Teeth If knocked out, handle the tooth by the top and not the root (the part that would be in the gum). If dirty, rinse gently with out scrubbing or touching the root. Do not use any cleansers. Use cold running water or milk. Place the tooth in clean water or milk and transport the tooth with the child when seeking emergency care. Call and go directly to the pediatric dentist or an emergency department. If the tooth is broken, save the pieces in milk and call the pediatric dentist right away. Stop bleeding using gauze or a cotton ball and pressure in the socket.

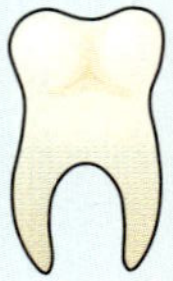

Stings, Bites, and Allergies

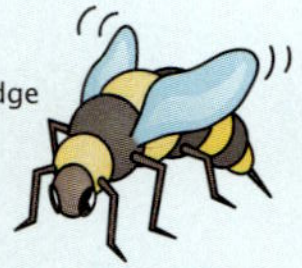

Stinging Insects Remove the stinger as soon as possible with a scraping motion using a firm item (such as the edge of a credit card). Put a cold compress on the bite to relieve the pain. If trouble breathing, fainting, or extreme swelling occurs, call 911 or an emergency number right away. For hives, nausea, or vomiting, call the pediatrician. For spider bites, call the pediatrician or Poison Center and describe the spider. Have the pediatrician check any bites that become infected.

Animal or Human Bites Wash wound well with soap and water. Call the pediatrician. The child may need a tetanus or rabies shot.

Ticks Use tweezers or your fingers to grasp as close as possible to the head of the tick and briskly pull the tick away from where it is attached. Call the pediatrician if the child develops symptoms such as a rash or fever.

Snake Bites Take the child to an emergency department if you are unsure of the type of snake or if you are concerned that the snake may be poisonous. Keep the child at rest. Do not apply ice. Loosely splint the injured area and keep it at rest, positioned at or slightly below the level of the heart. Identify the snake, if you can do so safely. If you are not able to identify the snake but are able to kill it safely, take it with you to the emergency department for identification.

Allergy Swelling, problems breathing, and paleness may be signs of severe allergy. Some people may have emergency medicine for these times. If possible, ask about emergency medicine they may have and help them administer it if necessary.

Skin Wounds

Make sure the child is up to date for tetanus vaccination. Any open wound may need a tetanus booster even when the child is currently immunized. If the child has an open wound, ask the pediatrician if the child needs a tetanus booster.

Bruises Apply cold compresses. Call the pediatrician if the child has a crush injury, large bruises, continued pain, or swelling. The pediatrician may recommend acetaminophen for pain.

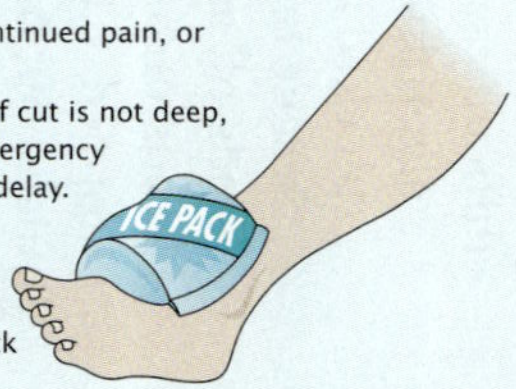

Cuts Rinse small cuts with water until clean. Use direct pressure with a clean cloth to stop bleeding. If cut is not deep, apply an antibiotic ointment, then cover the cut with a clean bandage. Call the pediatrician or seek emergency care for large and/or deep cuts, or if the wound is gaping, because stitches should be placed without delay. For major bleeding, call for help (911 or an emergency number). Continue direct pressure with a clean cloth until help arrives.

Scrapes Rinse with clean, running tap water for at least 5 minutes to remove dirt and germs. Do not use detergents, alcohol, or peroxide. Apply a triple antibiotic ointment and a bandage that will not stick to the wound.

Splinters Remove small splinters with tweezers, then wash and apply local antiseptic. If you cannot remove the splinter completely, call the pediatrician.

Puncture Wounds Do not remove large objects (such as a knife or stick) from a wound. Call for help (911 or an emergency number). Such objects must be removed by a doctor. Call the pediatrician for all puncture wounds. The child may need a tetanus booster.

Bleeding Apply pressure with gauze over the bleeding area. If still bleeding, add more gauze and apply pressure. Wrap an elastic bandage firmly over gauze and apply pressure. If bleeding continues, call the pediatrician or seek emergency care.

Burns and Scalds

General Treatment First stop the burning process by removing the child from contact with hot water or a hot object (for example, oil). If clothing is burning, smother flames and cool clothing by soaking with water. Remove clothing unless it is firmly stuck to the skin. Run cool water over burned skin until the pain stops. Do not apply ice, butter, grease, medicine, or ointment.

Burns With Blisters Do not break the blisters. Ask the pediatrician how to cover the burn and about burns on the face, hands, feet, or genitals.

Large or Deep Burns Call 911 or an emergency number. After stopping and cooling the burn, keep the child warm with a clean sheet covered with a blanket until help arrives.

Electrical Burns Disconnect electrical power. If the child is still in contact with electrical source, do **NOT** touch the child with bare hands. Pull the child away from the power source with an object that does not conduct electricity (such as a wooden pole), ***only after the power is turned off.*** **ALL** electrical burns need to be seen by a doctor.

Head Injuries

DO NOT MOVE A CHILD WHO MAY HAVE A SERIOUS HEAD, NECK, AND/OR BACK INJURY. This may cause further harm.

Call 911 or an emergency number right away if the child loses consciousness or has a convulsion (seizure).

Call the pediatrician for a child with a head injury and any of the following:

- Drowsiness
- Difficulty being awakened
- Persistent headache or vomiting
- Clumsiness or inability to move any body part
- Oozing of blood or watery fluid from ears or nose
- Abnormal speech or behavior

For any questions about less serious injuries, call the pediatrician.

Does your community have 911? If not, note the number of your local ambulance service and other important numbers below.

Be Prepared: Call 911

KEEP EMERGENCY NUMBERS BY YOUR TELEPHONE

PEDIATRICIAN ______________________

PEDIATRIC DENTIST ______________________

POISON CENTER 1-800-222-1222

AMBULANCE ______________________

EMERGENCY DEPARTMENT ______________________

FIRE ______________________

POLICE ______________________

DIRECTIONS TO THE LOCATION (ADDRESS, ETC, FOR BABYSITTERS, CAREGIVERS) ______________________

Turn Over for Choking and CPR Instructions

American Academy of Pediatrics

DEDICATED TO THE HEALTH OF ALL CHILDREN™

The information contained in this publication should not be used as a substitute for the medical care and advice of your pediatrician. There may be variations in treatment that your pediatrician may recommend based on individual facts and circumstances.

Index

T

U

V

W

Photo Credits

Chapter 1

Opener © David Young-Wolff/PhotoEdit

Chapter 2

Opener © SW Productions/Brand X Pictures/Getty Images; **Figure 2-2A** Courtesy of AAOS; **Figure 2-4** © St. Bartholomew's Hospital, London/Photo Researchers, Inc.

Chapter 3

Opener © David Young Wolff/PhotoEdit

Chapter 4

Opener © Stockbyte

Chapter 6

Opener © Medical-on-Line/Alamy Images

Chapter 8

Opener © Peter Adams/Index Stock Imagery; **Figure 8-2** Courtesy of Dey, L.P.

Chapter 9

Opener © Jonathan Plant/Alamy Images; **Figures 9-2A, 9-2B** Courtesy of Dr. Pratt/CDC; **Figure 9-2C** © Photos.com; **Figure 9-2D** Courtesy of Scott Bauer/USDA

Chapter 12

Opener © Catherine Dianich Grover/PhotoNations/Alamy Images

Chapter 13

Opener © Robert W. Ginn/PhotoEdit

Chapter 15

Opener © Say Cheese Company/Brand X Pictures/Getty Images; **Figure 15-1** © Creasource/PictureQuest; **Figure 15-2** © Jones and Bartlett Publishers. Photographed by Kimberly Potvin.

Unless otherwise indicated, photographs have been supplied by the Maryland Institute of Emergency Medical Service Systems.

Notes

Notes

Notes

Notes

Notes